Cutaneous Lymphomas

Editor

ANTONIO SUBTIL

SURGICAL PATHOLOGY CLINICS

surgpath.theclinics.com

Consulting Editor
JOHN R. GOLDBLUM

June 2014 • Volume 7 • Number 2

ELSEVIER

1600 John F. Kennedy Boulevard • Suite 1800 • Philadelphia, Pennsylvania, 19103-2899

http://www.theclinics.com

SURGICAL PATHOLOGY CLINICS Volume 7, Number 2
June 2014 ISSN 1875-9181, ISBN-13: 978-0-323-27784-6

Editor: Joanne Husovski
Developmental Editor: Donald Mumford

Surgical Pathology Clinics (ISSN 1875-9181) is published quarterly by Elsevier Inc., 360 Park Avenue South, New York, NY 10010. Months of issue are March, June, September, and December. Business and Editorial Office: Elsevier Inc., 1600 John F. Kennedy Blvd., Ste. 1800, Philadelphia, PA 19103-2899. Accounting and Circulation Offices: Elsevier Inc., 3251 Riverport Lane, Maryland Heights, MO 63043. Periodicals postage paid at New York, NY and at additional mailing offices. Subscription prices are $200.00 per year (US individuals), $233.00 per year (US institutions), $100.00 per year (US students/residents), $250.00 per year (Canadian individuals), $266.00 per year (Canadian Institutions), $250.00 per year (foreign individuals), $266.00 per year (foreign institutions), and $120.00 per year (international & Canadian students/residents). Foreign air speed delivery is included in all *Clinics'* subscription prices. All prices are subject to change without notice. **POSTMASTER:** Send address changes to *Surgical Pathology Clinics*, Elsevier, 3251 Riverport Lane, Maryland Heights, MO 63043. Customer Service: 1-800-654-2452 (US). From outside the United States, call 1-314-447-8871. Fax: 1-314-447-8029. E-mail: JournalsCustomerServiceusa@elsevier.com (for print support) and JournalsOnlineSupport-usa@elsevier.com (for online support).

Reprints. For copies of 100 or more, of articles in this publication, please contact the Commercial Reprints Department, Elsevier Inc., 360 Park Avenue South, New York, NY 10010-1710. Tel. 212-633-3874; Fax: 212-633-3820; E-mail: reprints@elsevier.com.

Contributors

CONSULTING EDITOR

JOHN R. GOLDBLUM, MD
Chairman, Professor of Pathology, Department
of Anatomic Pathology, Cleveland Clinics
Lerner College of Medicine, Cleveland Clinic,
Cleveland, Ohio

EDITOR

ANTONIO SUBTIL, MD, MBA
Associate Professor, Departments of
Dermatology and Pathology, Yale School of
Medicine; Board Certified, Dermatopathology
and Hematopathology, Yale Dermatopathology
Laboratory, Yale University, New Haven,
Connecticut

AUTHORS

BELÉN RUBIO GONZÁLEZ, MD
Dermatology Department, Hospital 12 de
Octubre, Madrid, Spain

JOAN GUITART, MD
Departments of Dermatology and Pathology,
Feinberg School of Medicine, Northwestern
University; Robert H. Lurie Comprehensive
Cancer Center, Chicago, Illinois

WERNER KEMPF, MD
Kempf und Pfaltz, Histologische Diagnostik;
Department of Dermatology, University
Hospital, Zürich, Switzerland

AGNIESZKA W. KUBICA, MD
Department of Dermatology, Mayo Clinic,
Rochester, Minnesota

M. ESTELA MARTÍNEZ-ESCALA, MD
Departments of Dermatology and Pathology,
Feinberg School of Medicine, Northwestern
University, Chicago, Illinois

LAURA B. PINCUS, MD
Assistant Professor of Dermatology and
Pathology, University of California, San
Francisco, San Francisco, California

MARK R. PITTELKOW, MD
Department of Dermatology, Mayo Clinic,
Scottsdale, Arizona

ANTONIO SUBTIL, MD, MBA
Associate Professor, Departments of
Dermatology and Pathology, Yale School of
Medicine; Board Certified, Dermatopathology
and Hematopathology, Yale Dermatopathology
Laboratory, Yale University, New Haven,
Connecticut

UMA SUNDRAM, MD, PhD
Assistant Professor, Departments of Pathology
and Dermatology, Stanford Hospital and
Clinics, Stanford, California

REIN WILLEMZE, MD
Department of Dermatology, Leiden University
Medical Center, Leiden, The Netherlands

Contents

Both pathology and dermatology rely heavily on a visual approach to learning, generating differential diagnoses, and making diagnoses. Pattern recognition and the development of diagnostic frameworks are essential elements in this process. In addition to images, several algorithms and summaries are presented in this article to provide a practical approach to the diagnosis of cutaneous lymphoproliferative disorders. The critical importance of clinical pathologic correlation is also emphasized.

This article is a comprehensive review of mycosis fungoides (MF), the most common type of cutaneous T-cell lymphoma. The first portion of the article introduces epidemiologic features of MF. Next, the clinical presentation is described, followed by the microscopic features. This article addresses how to establish a diagnosis of MF and includes a discussion of the utility of ancillary testing, such as immunohistochemistry and T-cell clonality testing. The differential diagnosis is also discussed, with attention to how to distinguish MF from histopathologic mimics. The final section of the article discusses prognosis and risk of disease progression in MF.

Mycosis fungoides (MF) is a cutaneous T-cell lymphoma that usually manifests as patches and plaques with a propensity for nonphotoexposed areas. MF is a common mimicker of inflammatory and infectious skin diseases, because it can be manifested with a wide variety of clinical and pathologic presentations. These atypical presentations of MF may be difficult to diagnose, requiring a high level of suspicion and careful clinicopathologic correlation. Within this array of clinical presentations, the World Health Organization classification recognizes 3 MF variants: folliculotropic MF, pagetoid reticulosis, and granulomatous slack skin. These 3 variants, as well as hypopigmented MF, are addressed in this article.

Sézary syndrome (SS), a type of cutaneous T-cell lymphoma with a poor prognosis, is characterized by erythroderma and leukemic involvement. Because of the rarity of SS and difficulty in diagnosis, data on this aggressive malignancy are scarce. In this review, the diagnosis and pathology of SS are summarized and an update is provided, highlighting microscopic features and novel molecular findings. The diagnostic challenge of SS is described, with an emphasis on the differential diagnosis of erythroderma and key points in distinguishing SS from other cutaneous T-cell malignancies. Finally, the prognosis is discussed, focusing on large, recent studies of SS patients.

Cutaneous CD30+ lymphoproliferative disorders are the second most common types of cutaneous T-cell lymphomas. They represent a well-defined spectrum encompassing lymphomatoid papulosis (LyP), primary cutaneous anaplastic large-cell lymphoma (pcALCL), and borderline lesions. They share the expression of CD30 as a common phenotypic hallmark, but they differ in their clinical presentation, course, and histologic features. New variants have been recently identified, including CD8+ epidermotropic LyP type D, angioinvasive LyP type E, and ALK-positive pcALCL. This review describes clinical, histopathologic, and phenotypic variants; their differential diagnoses (benign and malignant); and the role of CD30 as a diagnostic, prognostic, and therapeutic marker.

Primary cutaneous T-cell lymphomas (CTCLs), other than mycosis fungoides/Sézary syndrome and the group of cutaneous CD30+ lymphoproliferative disorders, are rare. These include subcutaneous panniculitis–like T-cell lymphoma (SPTCL); extranodal natural killer/T-cell lymphoma, nasal type; primary cutaneous peripheral T-cell lymphoma, not otherwise specified (PTCL, NOS); and rare subtypes of PTCL, NOS. Apart from SPTCL and primary cutaneous CD4-positive small-medium pleomorphic T-cell lymphoma, these lymphomas have in common aggressive clinical behavior and poor prognosis. Differentiation between these different types of CTCL may be difficult and requires integration of histopathologic findings with clinical data and the results of phenotypic and often molecular genetic studies.

Primary cutaneous B cell lymphomas (PCBCL) are rare and tend to be indolent disorders, with one exception, that of primary cutaneous diffuse large B cell lymphoma-leg type. In indolent conditions, the distinction between cutaneous lymphoma and cutaneous lymphoid hyperplasia can be difficult, on histopathologic, immunohistochemical and even molecular grounds. Integration of all available information, including the clinical setting, is crucial to arriving at the appropriate diagnosis. In this review we will cover the diagnostic approaches to primary cutaneous marginal zone lymphoma, primary cutaneous follicle center lymphoma, and primary cutaneous diffuse large B cell lymphoma-leg type, and discuss their differential diagnosis.

SURGICAL PATHOLOGY CLINICS

Preface
Pathology of Cutaneous Lymphomas

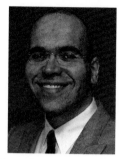

Antonio Subtil, MD, MBA
Editor

Our knowledge of cutaneous lymphomas has been significantly growing as a result of important discoveries in immunology, molecular biology, and immunohistochemistry. In addition, improved clinical pathologic correlation and follow-up data, as well as the synergistic collaboration among different lymphoma registries and specialists from several academic medical centers in order to study rare variants, have greatly contributed to the understanding of the difficult field of cutaneous lymphoproliferative disorders. While these advances have increased our knowledge of skin lymphomas, they have also produced an extensive and sometimes confusing litany of articles, studies, and classification schemes. This issue on "Cutaneous Lymphomas" in *Surgical Pathology Clinics* provides an organized and updated review of this challenging topic by internationally recognized experts and bridges critical knowledge gaps in the diagnosis of cutaneous lymphomas. Both common and rare entities are reviewed. The article by Pincus covers the most common type of skin lymphoma: mycosis fungoides (MF). Unique clinicopathologic variants of MF are reviewed in the article by Martinez-Escala et al, and Sézary syndrome in the article by Kubica and Pittelkow. The article by Kempf reviews the spectrum of cutaneous CD30-positive lymphoproliferative disorders. The article by Willemze covers the heterogeneous group of T-cell lymphomas without clinical features of MF or CD30 expression. Finally, cutaneous B-cell lymphomas are reviewed in the article by Sundram. In addition to multiple clinical and microscopic images, several tables and algorithms are presented to aid in diagnosis and staging. Beyond its usefulness to general pathologists, dermatopathologists, and hematopathologists, this information is intended to be helpful for dermatologists, hematologists/oncologists, fellows, and residents.

I would like to acknowledge and thank Dr. John Goldblum for inviting me to be a guest editor, and Joanne Husovski for her support and outstanding editor skills.

Antonio Subtil, MD, MBA
Associate Professor
Departments of Dermatology and Pathology
Board Certified
Dermatopathology and Hematopathology
Yale University School of Medicine
15 York Street, LMP 5031
New Haven, CT 06520, USA

E-mail address:
antonio.subtil@yale.edu

Surgical Pathology 7 (2014) ix
http://dx.doi.org/10.1016/j.path.2014.02.008
1875-9181/14/$ – see front matter © 2014 Elsevier Inc. All rights reserved.

A General Approach to the Diagnosis of Cutaneous Lymphomas and Pseudolymphomas

Antonio Subtil, MD, MBA

KEYWORDS

- Cutaneous lymphomas • Pseudolymphomas • Skin • T-cell • B-cell • Lymphoma • Diagnosis
- Histopathology • Dermis • Epidermis

KEY POINTS

- Both pathology and dermatology rely heavily on a visual approach to learning, generating differential diagnoses (DDx), and making diagnoses.
- Pattern recognition and the development of diagnostic frameworks are essential elements in this process.
- In addition to images, several tables and algorithms are presented in this article to provide a practical approach to the diagnosis of cutaneous lymphoproliferative disorders.
- The critical importance of clinical pathologic correlation is also emphasized.

ABSTRACT

Both pathology and dermatology rely heavily on a visual approach to learning, generating differential diagnoses, and making diagnoses. Pattern recognition and the development of diagnostic frameworks are essential elements in this process. In addition to images, several algorithms and summaries are presented in this article to provide a practical approach to the diagnosis of cutaneous lymphoproliferative disorders. The critical importance of clinical pathologic correlation is also emphasized.

updated review of this challenging topic by an international team of experts and bridges critical knowledge gaps in the diagnosis of cutaneous lymphomas. In addition to multiple clinical and microscopic images, several tables are presented to aid in diagnosis and staging. Both common and rare entities are reviewed—mycosis fungoides (MF), unique clinicopathologic variants of MF, cutaneous CD30-positive lymphoproliferative disorders, T-cell lymphomas without clinical features of MF or CD30 expression, and cutaneous B-cell lymphomas. For all entities, careful correlation of clinical and histopathologic findings is essential to arrive at the correct diagnosis (Fig. 1).

Considering the heterogeneity and complexity of cutaneous lymphoproliferative disorders,[1–3] this introductory article includes several tables and algorithms to provide a practical and logical approach to DDx based on different clinical

OVERVIEW

This issue on "Cutaneous Lymphomas" in *Surgical Pathology Clinics* provides an organized and

Disclosure Statement: No financial disclosures or conflicts of interest.
Yale Dermatopathology Laboratory, Yale School of Medicine, 15 York Street, LMP 5031, New Haven, CT 06520-8059, USA
E-mail address: antonio.subtil@yale.edu

Surgical Pathology 7 (2014) 135–142
http://dx.doi.org/10.1016/j.path.2014.02.007
1875-9181/14/$ – see front matter © 2014 Elsevier Inc. All rights reserved.

Clinical + Path = Diagnosis

*Clinical pathologic correlation is essential to
diagnose skin lymphoma*

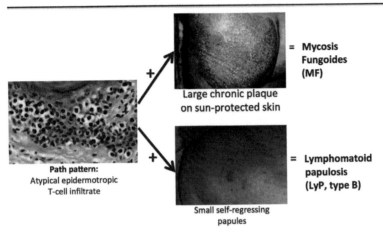

Path pattern:
Atypical epidermotropic
T-cell infiltrate

+   Large chronic plaque
on sun-protected skin

= **Mycosis
Fungoides
(MF)**

+   Small self-regressing
papules

= **Lymphomatoid
papulosis
(LyP, type B)**

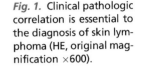

Fig. 1. Clinical pathologic
correlation is essential to
the diagnosis of skin lymphoma (HE, original mag-
nification ×600).

findings (**Fig. 2**, **Table 1**) and histopathologic patterns (**Boxes 1–6**, **Figs. 3–7**). Within the differential
list, each diagnostic possibility includes a link to a
corresponding article for further information. In addition, it is important to recognize that several
diseases (benign and malignant) may mimic cuta-
neous lymphomas. A comprehensive list of pseudolymphomas is provided in **Box 7**.

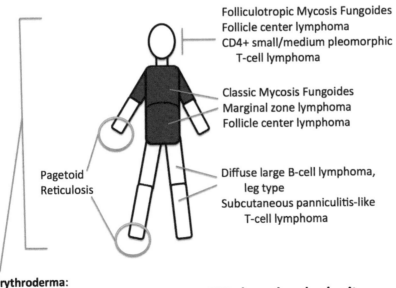

Folliculotropic Mycosis Fungoides
Follicle center lymphoma
CD4+ small/medium pleomorphic
T-cell lymphoma

Classic Mycosis Fungoides
Marginal zone lymphoma
Follicle center lymphoma

Pagetoid
Reticulosis

Diffuse large B-cell lymphoma,
leg type
Subcutaneous panniculitis-like
T-cell lymphoma

Erythroderma:
Sézary syndrome

DDx based on body site

Fig. 2. DDx based on body
site.

Table 1
Differential diagnosis based on the provided clinical information

If the Clinical Information Is…	Consider…
Long history of large patches and/or plaques on sun-protected skin	MF See the article by Pincus elsewhere in this issue.
Alopecia and/or follicular-based lesions	Folliculotropic MF See the article by Martinez-Escala and colleagues elsewhere in this issue.
Erythroderma (>80% of total body erythema)	Sézary syndrome See the article by Kubica and Pittelkow elsewhere in this issue.
Several small self-regressing lesions	Lymphomatoid papulosis See the article by Kempf elsewhere in this issue.
Rapid onset and progression of multiple, ulcerated, nonregressing skin lesions	Primary cutaneous CD8+ aggressive epidermotropic cytotoxic T-cell lymphoma, cutaneous gamma/delta T-cell lymphoma, extranodal natural killer/T-cell lymphoma, nasal type See the article by Willemze elsewhere in this issue.
Solitary or grouped plaques and tumors on the scalp or on the back	Primary cutaneous follicle center lymphoma See the article by Sundram elsewhere in this issue.
Solitary or multifocal papules, plaques, or nodules on the trunk and arms	Primary cutaneous marginal zone lymphoma See the article by Sundram elsewhere in this issue.
Rapidly growing tumors on one or both (lower) legs of elderly patient	Primary cutaneous diffuse large B-cell lymphoma, leg type See the article by Sundram elsewhere in this issue.

Box 1
Differential diagnosis of large cell lymphoid infiltrate (>25%–30% large cells)

- Large cell transformation of MF

    See the article by Pincus elsewhere in this issue.

- LyP type C

    The histologic features of LyP type C and pcALCL as well as sALCL are identical. To separate these entities, integration of clinical presentation and staging results as well as phenotypic and genetic findings are mandatory. See the article by Kempf elsewhere in this issue.

- Cutaneous anaplastic large cell lymphoma

    See the article by Kempf elsewhere in this issue.

- Some cases of aggressive cytotoxic cutaneous lymphomas

    See the article by Willemze elsewhere in this issue.

- Primary cutaneous peripheral T-cell lymphoma, unspecified

    See the article by Willemze elsewhere in this issue.

- Primary cutaneous diffuse large B-cell lymphoma, leg type

    See the article by Sundram elsewhere in this issue.

Abbreviations: LyP, lymphomatoid papulosis; pcALCL, primary cutaneous anaplastic large cell lymphoma; sALCL, systemic anaplastic large cell lymphoma.

Box 2
Differential diagnosis of perifollicular accentuation (lymphoid infiltrate around hair follicles)

- Folliculotropic MF

    See the article by Martinez-Escala and colleagues elsewhere in this issue.

- Primary cutaneous marginal zone lymphoma

    See the article by Sundram elsewhere in this issue.

- Some cases of lymphomatoid papulosis

    See the article by Kempf elsewhere in this issue.

- Cutaneous pseudolymphoma: herpes folliculitis, pseudolymphomatous folliculitis, persistent arthropod bite reactions (see **Box 7**)

Box 3
Differential diagnosis of cutaneous lymphoid infiltrate with frequent eosinophils

- Folliculotropic MF

    See the article by Martinez-Escala and colleagues elsewhere in this issue.

- Lymphomatoid papulosis type A

    See the article by Kempf elsewhere in this issue.

- Cutaneous pseudolymphoma: lymphomatoid drug eruption, persistent arthropod bite reactions, scabies, exaggerated bitelike reactions in the setting of systemic hematologic disorders (see **Box 7**)

Box 4
Differential diagnosis of CD8 expression

- Lymphomatoid papulosis type D

    See the article by Kempf elsewhere in this issue.

- Some cases of otherwise classical MF

    See the article by Pincus elsewhere in this issue.

- Many cases of pagetoid reticulosis

    See the article by Martinez-Escala and colleagues elsewhere in this issue.

- Some cases of cutaneous anaplastic large cell lymphoma

    See the article by Kempf elsewhere in this issue.

- Primary cutaneous CD8$^+$ aggressive epidermotropic cytotoxic T-cell lymphoma

    See the article by Willemze elsewhere in this issue.

- Subcutaneous panniculitis-like T-cell lymphoma

    See the article by Willemze elsewhere in this issue.

- Many cases of cutaneous gamma/delta T-cell lymphoma

    See the article by Willemze elsewhere in this issue.

- Indolent CD8$^+$ lymphoid proliferation of the ear

    See the article by Willemze elsewhere in this issue.

- Cutaneous pseudolymphoma: CD8$^+$ infiltrates in the setting of advanced AIDS (see **Box 7**)

Box 5
Differential diagnosis of CD30 expression

- Lymphomatoid papulosis

    See the article by Kempf elsewhere in this issue.

- Cutaneous anaplastic large cell lymphoma

    See the article by Kempf elsewhere in this issue.

- Many (but not all) cases of large cell transformation of MF

    See the article by Pincus elsewhere in this issue.

- Some cases of folliculotropic MF and pagetoid reticulosis

    See the article by Martinez-Escala and colleagues elsewhere in this issue.

- Some cases of aggressive cytotoxic cutaneous lymphomas

    See the article by Willemze elsewhere in this issue.

- Cutaneous pseudolymphoma: reactive lymphoid hyperplasia in the setting of viral infection, persistent arthropod bite reactions and scabies (see Box 7)

Box 6
Scenarios to consider: Epstein-Barr virus in situ hybridization (Epstein-Barr virus encoded small RNA)

- Presence of angiocentrism/angiodestruction
- Presence of extensive, infarct-like necrosis
- Cytotoxic immunophenotype
- Prominent CD56 expression
- Presence of both skin and lung lesions
- Young patients with facial edema
- Elderly patients
- Immunodeficiency
- History of transplant

Abbreviations: EBER, Epstein-Barr virus Encoded small RNA; EBV, Epstein-Barr virus.

Fig. 3. DDx of epidermotropism (HE, original magnification ×600).

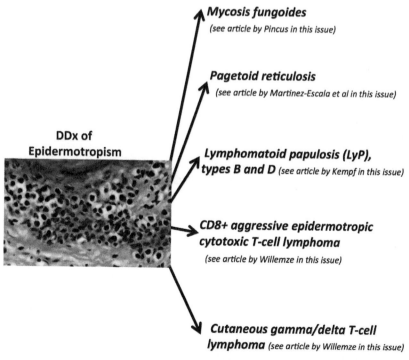

DDx of Epidermotropism

Mycosis fungoides
(see article by Pincus in this issue)

Pagetoid reticulosis
(see article by Martinez-Escala et al in this issue)

Lymphomatoid papulosis (LyP), types B and D *(see article by Kempf in this issue)*

CD8+ aggressive epidermotropic cytotoxic T-cell lymphoma
(see article by Willemze in this issue)

Cutaneous gamma/delta T-cell lymphoma *(see article by Willemze in this issue)*

DDx of Ulceration

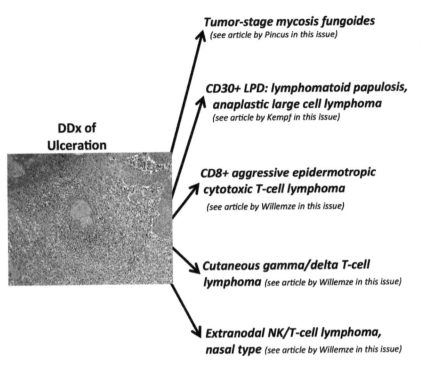

Tumor-stage mycosis fungoides
(see article by Pincus in this issue)

CD30+ LPD: lymphomatoid papulosis, anaplastic large cell lymphoma
(see article by Kempf in this issue)

CD8+ aggressive epidermotropic cytotoxic T-cell lymphoma
(see article by Willemze in this issue)

Cutaneous gamma/delta T-cell lymphoma *(see article by Willemze in this issue)*

Extranodal NK/T-cell lymphoma, nasal type *(see article by Willemze in this issue)*

Fig. 4. DDx of ulceration (HE, original magnification ×400).

DDx of prominent lymphoid follicles

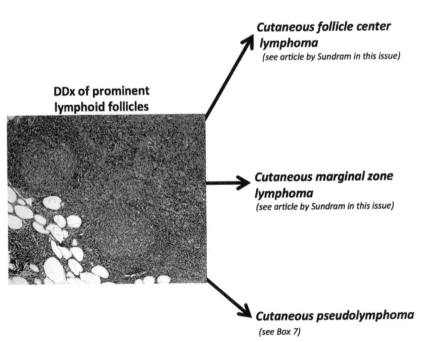

Cutaneous follicle center lymphoma
(see article by Sundram in this issue)

Cutaneous marginal zone lymphoma
(see article by Sundram in this issue)

Cutaneous pseudolymphoma
(see Box 7)

Fig. 5. DDx of a cutaneous lymphoid infiltrate with prominent lymphoid follicles (HE, original magnification ×200).

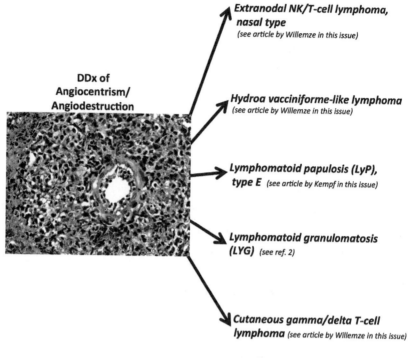

Fig. 6. DDx of a cutaneous lymphoid infiltrate with angiocentrism and angio-destruction (HE, original magnification ×400).

DDx of Angiocentrism/ Angiodestruction

Extranodal NK/T-cell lymphoma, nasal type
(see article by Willemze in this issue)

Hydroa vacciniforme-like lymphoma
(see article by Willemze in this issue)

Lymphomatoid papulosis (LyP), type E *(see article by Kempf in this issue)*

Lymphomatoid granulomatosis (LYG) *(see ref. 2)*

Cutaneous gamma/delta T-cell lymphoma *(see article by Willemze in this issue)*

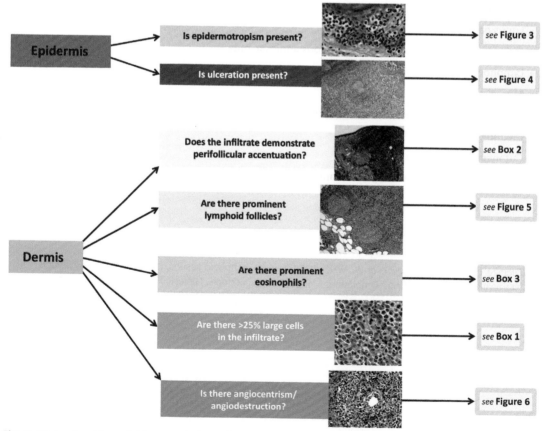

Epidermis

Is epidermotropism present? → *see* **Figure 3**

Is ulceration present? → *see* **Figure 4**

Dermis

Does the infiltrate demonstrate perifollicular accentuation? → *see* **Box 2**

Are there prominent lymphoid follicles? → *see* **Figure 5**

Are there prominent eosinophils? → *see* **Box 3**

Are there >25% large cells in the infiltrate? → *see* **Box 1**

Is there angiocentrism/ angiodestruction? → *see* **Figure 6**

Fig. 7. Basic algorithm of histomorphologic findings in the epidermis and dermis for cutaneous lymphoid infiltrates.

Box 7
Cutaneous pseudolymphomas (histopathologic mimics of skin lymphoma)

- Lymphomatoid drug eruption
- Reactive lymphoid hyperplasia in the setting of viral infection (herpes folliculitis, inflamed molluscum contagiosum, orf, or milker's nodule)
- Cutaneous leishmaniasis
- Syphilis
- *Borrelia* infection
- Persistent nodular scabies
- Persistent arthropod bite reactions
- Exaggerated bitelike reactions in the setting of systemic hematologic disorders
- Pseudolymphomatous tattoo reaction
- Reactive lymphoid hyperplasia at sites of vaccination
- Inflammatory stage of vitiligo
- Early stage of lichen sclerosus et atrophicus
- Inflammatory stage of morphea
- Lymphomatoid lichenoid keratosis
- Pigmented purpuric dermatoses
- Pityriasis lichenoides
- Lupus panniculitis
- Pseudolymphomatous variant of cutaneous angiosarcoma
- Lymphoepithelioma-like carcinoma of the skin
- Merkel cell carcinoma
- Acral pseudolymphomatous angiokeratoma of children (APACHE)
- Pseudolymphomatous folliculitis
- Cutaneous plasmacytosis
- CD8+ infiltrates in the setting of advanced AIDS

REFERENCES

1. Willemze R, Jaffe ES, Burg G, et al. WHO-EORTC classification for cutaneous lymphomas. Blood 2005;105:3768–85.

2. Swerdlow SH, Campo E, Harris NL, et al, editors. WHO classification of tumors of hematopoietic and lymphoid tissues. Lyon (France): IARC; 2008.

3. Cerroni L, Gatter K, Kerl H. Skin lymphoma: the illustrated guide. Oxford (United Kingdom): Wiley-Blackwell; 2009.

Mycosis Fungoides

Laura B. Pincus, MD

KEYWORDS

- Mycosis fungoides • Cutaneous T-cell lymphoma • Skin lymphoma • Cutaneous oncology

KEY POINTS

- The histopathology of patch-stage mycosis fungoides (MF) is characterized by patchy to well-developed bandlike infiltrates of small to medium-sized lymphocytes within the papillary dermis combined with epidermotropism of lymphocytes and fibrosis of the papillary dermis.
- Plaque-stage disease has features similar to patch-stage disease, but the infiltrate is often denser and extends into the reticular dermis. Epidermotropism is usually more marked.
- Tumor-stage disease is characterized by dense and diffuse infiltrates of atypical lymphocytes in the reticular dermis that often extend into the subcutaneous tissue. Epidermotropism may be absent.
- The above-described histopathology in all stages is not specific for MF, because similar features are seen in other conditions. Therefore, establishing a diagnosis of MF requires integration of the clinical presentation with the histopathology.

ABSTRACT

This article is a comprehensive review of mycosis fungoides (MF), the most common type of cutaneous T-cell lymphoma. The first portion of the article introduces epidemiologic features of MF. Next, the clinical presentation is described, followed by the microscopic features. This article addresses how to establish a diagnosis of MF and includes a discussion of the utility of ancillary testing, such as immunohistochemistry and T-cell clonality testing. The differential diagnosis is also discussed, with attention to how to distinguish MF from histopathologic mimics. The final section of the article discusses prognosis and risk of disease progression in MF.

lymphoma composed of epidermotropic infiltrates of neoplastic T lymphocytes. It occurs more frequently in older adults, with a median age at presentation reported between 57 and 61 years.[2,3] Nonetheless, a sizable number of cases occur in children. MF affects men more than women, with a ratio of approximately 2:1.[1] The incidence of MF has been estimated at 0.36 cases per 100,000 people per year[4] and seems to be increasing,[5] although this number has been difficult to determine because the distinction between MF and other forms of CTCL has not been consistent in different tumor registries. The condition seems more common in blacks than whites.[6] Although speculated as caused by an infectious agent, the etiology of the condition remains unknown.

OVERVIEW

MF is the most common type of cutaneous T-cell lymphoma (CTCL), constituting approximately 50% of all cases.[1] It is a primary cutaneous

CLINICAL FEATURES

The 3 main stages of cutaneous involvement of MF include patch-, plaque-, and tumor-stage disease (erythroderma is uncommon and is discussed in

Disclosure Statement: The author has no disclosures or no conflicts of interest.
Departments of Dermatology and Pathology, Section of Dermatopathology, University of California, San Francisco, 1701 Divisadero Street, Suite 280, San Francisco, CA 94115, USA
E-mail address: Laura.Pincus@ucsf.edu

Surgical Pathology 7 (2014) 143–167
http://dx.doi.org/10.1016/j.path.2014.02.004
1875-9181/14/$ – see front matter © 2014 Elsevier Inc. All rights reserved.

greater detail in an article by Kubica and Pittelkow). In all stages of disease, typical sites of involvement include photo-protected areas, in particular the buttocks, groin, breasts, upper thighs, and axilla and, less commonly, the distal extremities, head, and neck. In patch-stage disease, lesions are typically erythematous patches without significant induration or elevation and with fine overlying scale. Lesions are usually round, are between 5 and 10 cm in diameter (Figs. 1–3), and frequently have a wrinkled appearance, which is probably correlated with loss of elastic fibers (Figs. 4 and 5). Plaques are usually the same size and shape as patches but are

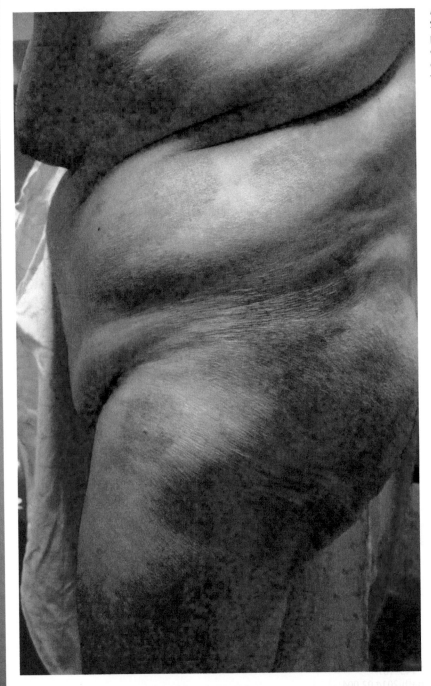

Fig. 1. MF, patch stage. Subtle large erythematous patches widely distributed on sun-protected sites, including the flanks, buttocks, and upper thighs.

Fig. 2. MF, patch stage. Detail of large erythematous patches on the flank.

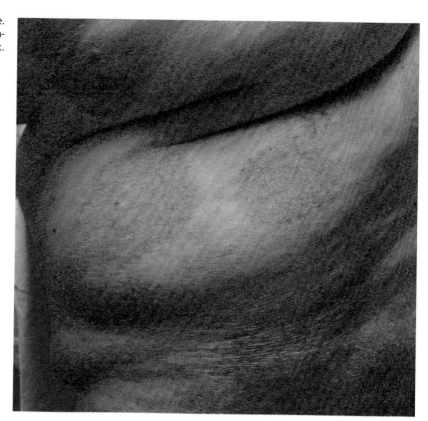

thicker than patches, because induration and/or elevation is present. Plaques are either round or annular and typically occur in continuity with patches (**Figs. 6–8**). Tumors usually develop within patches and/or plaques and present as nodules that are at least 1 cm in diameter (**Figs. 9–11**).[7] Although all patients with tumor-stage disease have progressed invariably from patch/plaque

Fig. 3. MF, patch stage. The buttocks are a frequent site of involvement, as in this case.

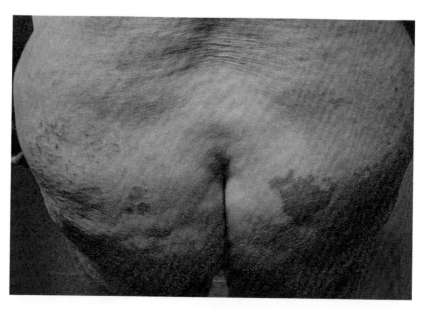

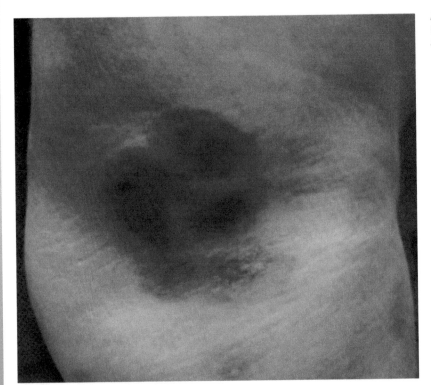

Fig. 4. MF, patch stage. Patch with a fine-wrinkled appearance.

disease, many patients with patch- or plaque-stage disease never progress to tumor stage.

Many clinical variants of MF have the same prognosis as conventional MF and, therefore, are not considered clinically meaningful variants in the current World Health Organization classification system for cutaneous lymphomas.[1] Such variants include acanthosis nigricans–like MF, dyshidrotic MF, and hypopigmented MF, which is a variant frequently seen in children.[8] However,

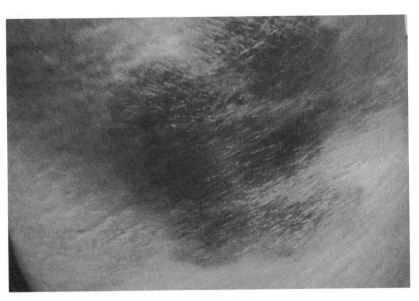

Fig. 5. MF, patch stage. Detail of patch with a fine-wrinkled appearance.

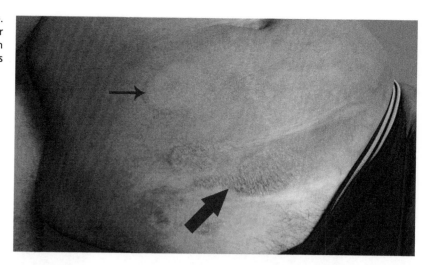

Fig. 6. MF, plaque stage. Plaques on the lower abdomen (*thick arrow*) in combination with patches (*thin arrow*).

there are some variants with distinct clinical and pathologic features which are considered clinically meaning in the current classification system, and these variants are discussed in detail in an article by Martinez-Escala and collegues.

Extracutaneous involvement may occur in late-stage disease, although it is rare. Sites of spread include the blood, lymph nodes, spleen, and liver.[1] See **Tables 1** and **2** for details of staging.

DIAGNOSIS: MICROSCOPIC FEATURES

Patch-stage disease is characterized by a patchy, bandlike infiltrate of small to medium-sized lymphocytes within the superficial dermis along with epidermal acanthosis and fibrosis in the papillary dermis (**Figs. 12** and **13**). Although the infiltrate may be sparse, the combination of the above-mentioned features with the presence of lymphocytes within the epidermis, also known as epidermotropism, in the absence of concomitant spongiosis, is characteristic of early disease (**Figs. 14–16**).[9] In more developed lesions, the infiltrate is often more dense, forming a well-developed bandlike lichenoid infiltrate of lymphocytes (**Fig. 17**), and epidermotropism is often more obvious (**Fig. 18**).

Epidermotropism is present in approximately 96% of cases.[10] One form of epidermotropism consists of large intraepidermal collections of lymphocytes, known as Pautrier microabscesses (**Fig. 19**). Although these collections are fairly

Fig. 7. MF, plaque stage. Patches and plaques in groin region, which is a typical location for MF.

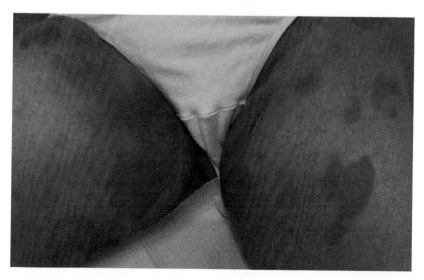

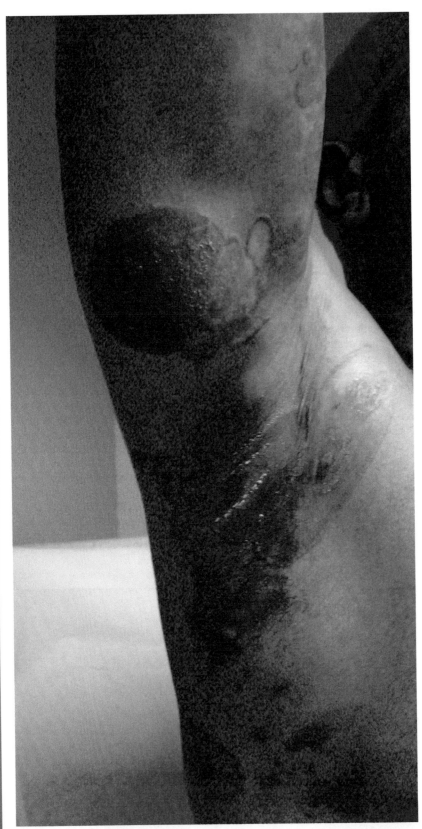

Fig. 8. MF, plaque stage. Plaques with an annular configuration and a raised border.

Fig. 9. MF, tumor stage. Tumors amid patches and plaques on the upper legs.

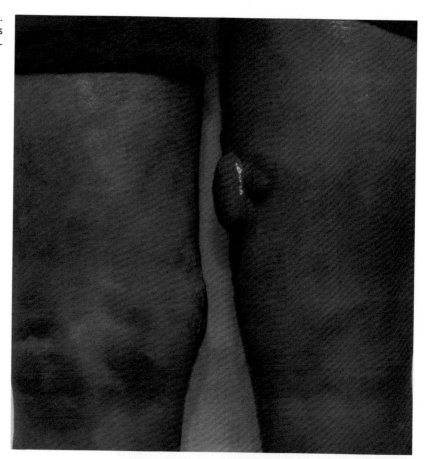

Key Features
MYCOSIS FUNGOIDES

Clinical

- Patch stage: erythematous patches with fine overlying scale that are usually at least 5 cm in diameter. Typically involve photo-protected sites.

- Plaque stage: lesions are the same size and shape as patches and involve the same sites but are thicker, displaying induration and/or elevation. Plaques are usually adjacent to patches.

- Tumor stage: lesions are at least 1 cm in diameter and are solid nodules with evidence of vertical growth. They usually develop within patches and plaques.

Histopathology

- Patch stage: patchy to well-developed bandlike infiltrates of small to medium-sized lymphocytes within the superficial dermis combined with epidermotropism of lymphocytes and fibrosis of the papillary dermis.

- Plaque stage: features similar to patch-stage disease, but the infiltrate is often denser and extends into the reticular dermis. Epidermotropism usually more marked.

- Tumor stage: dense and diffuse infiltrates of atypical lymphocytes in the reticular dermis that often extend into the subcutaneous tissue. Admixed eosinophils, plasma cells, and histiocytes are often present. Epidermotropism may be absent.

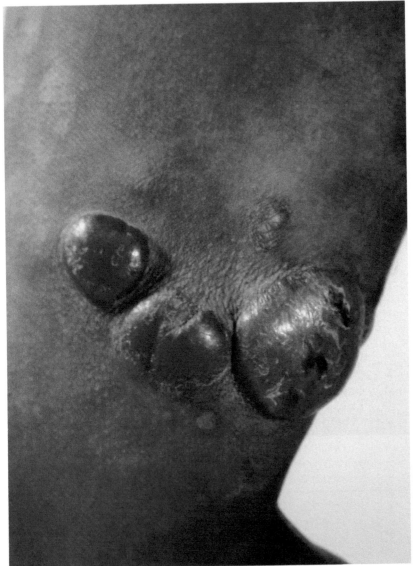

Fig. 10. MF, tumor stage. Detailed view of tumors.

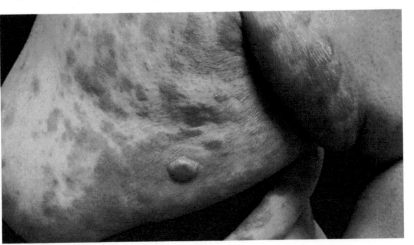

Fig. 11. MF, tumor stage. Tumors amid patches and plaques on the lateral breast.

Table 1
International Society for Cutaneous Lymphomas/European Organisation for Research and Treatment of Cancer revision to the classification of mycosis fungoides

Skin

T1	Patches and plaques covering <10% body surface area
T2	Patches and plaques covering >10% body surface area
T3	At least 1 tumor
T4	Erythroderma involving at least 80% body surface area

Lymph node

N0	No clinically abnormal peripheral lymph nodes
N1	Clinically abnormal peripheral lymph nodes; histopathology Dutch grade 1 or NCI LN0-2
N2	Clinically abnormal peripheral lymph nodes; histopathology Dutch grade 2 or NCI LN3
N3	Clinically abnormal peripheral lymph nodes; histopathology Dutch grades 3–4 or NCI LN4
NX	Clinically abnormal peripheral lymph nodes; no histologic confirmation

Visceral

M0	No visceral organ involvement
M1	Visceral involvement

Blood

B0	Absence of significant blood involvement
B1	Low tumor burden: >5% of peripheral blood lymphocytes are atypical cells but does not meet the criteria of B_2
B2	High tumor burden: $\geq$1000 μL Sézary cells with positive clone

Data from Olsen E, Vonderheid E, Pimpinelli N, et al. Revisions to the staging and classification of mycosis fungoides and Sézary syndrome: a proposal of the International Society for Cutaneous Lymphomas (ISCL) and the cutaneous lymphoma task force of the European Organization of Research and Treatment of Cancer (EORTC). Blood 2007;110:1713–22.

Table 2
International Society for Cutaneous Lymphomas/European Organisation for Research and Treatment of Cancer revision to the staging of mycosis fungoides

	T	N	M	B
IA	1	0	0	0, 1
IB	2	0	0	0, 1
II	1, 2	1, 2	0	0, 1
IIB	3	0–2	0	0, 1
IIIA	4	0–2	0	0
IIIB	4	0–2	0	1
IVA1	1–4	0–2	0	2
IVA2	1–4	3	0	0–2
IVB	1–4	0–3	1	0–2

Data from Olsen E, Vonderheid E, Pimpinelli N, et al. Revisions to the staging and classification of mycosis fungoides and Sézary syndrome: a proposal of the International Society for Cutaneous Lymphomas (ISCL) and the cutaneous lymphoma task force of the European Organization of Research and Treatment of Cancer (EORTC). Blood 2007;110:1713–22.

specific for MF, they are infrequently present. Other patterns include intraepidermal lymphocytes arranged as single cells, lymphocytes aligned along the basal layer of the epidermis (**Figs. 20** and **21**), haloed lymphocytes (individual lymphocytes surrounded by a cleft), and a disproportionate number of lymphocytes within the epidermis in the absence of spongiosis.[10] The presence of lymphocytes within the epidermis that are slightly larger than those in the dermis is a helpful diagnostic clue as well (**Fig. 22**). The lesional lymphocytes are not usually atypical (only 9% in a recent study)[9,10] and reactive lymphocytes are admixed with neoplastic lymphocytes.[11] Therefore, the diagnosis often rests more on architectural abnormalities than on cytologic atypicality.[12]

Plaque-stage disease is characterized by a denser bandlike infiltrate and extension of the infiltrate into the reticular dermis (**Fig. 23**). The epidermotropism is often more developed (**Figs. 24–26**)[13] and cytologic atypia is often more pronounced (**Fig. 27**). Most of the lesional cells are neoplastic, and thus the diagnosis is often easier to render than in early patch-stage disease.[14]

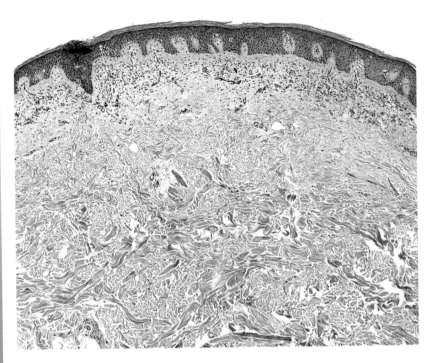

Fig. 12. MF, early patch stage. A patchy, bandlike infiltrate of small to medium-sized lymphocytes is present within the superficial dermis. The overlying epidermis is often acanthotic, and fibrosis is typically present in the papillary dermis. A subtle focus of epidermotropism is present (*arrow*) (HE, original magnification ×100).

Tumor-stage disease is typified by dense and diffuse infiltrates of often atypical-appearing lymphocytes in the reticular dermis and subcutis (**Figs. 28** and **29**). Mitotic figures can be identified (**Fig. 30**). Admixed eosinophils, plasma cells, and histiocytes are often present.[13] The epidermis is often ulcerated (**Fig. 31**). Epidermotropism may be absent.[1]

In large cell transformation, more than 25% of lesional cells are large and may form microscopic nodules (**Fig. 32**).[15] Large cell transformation occurs most frequently in tumor-stage disease, although it can also occur in patch/plaque stage. Atypical mitotic figures are often evident among the atypical lymphocytes (**Fig. 33**). CD30 expression may or may not be identified.[16]

Fig. 13. MF, early patch stage. Fibrosis of the papillary dermis (HE, original magnification ×200).

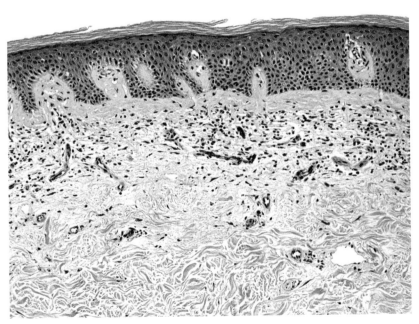

Fig. 14. MF, early patch stage. Subtle foci of epidermotropism of lesional lymphocytes (HE, original magnification ×400).

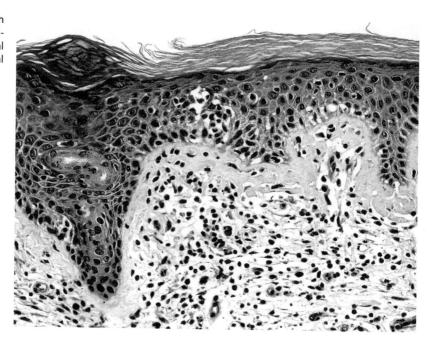

DIAGNOSIS: ANCILLARY STUDIES

In most cases, the lesional cells in early MF display a CD3$^+$/CD4$^+$/CD8$^-$/CD45RO$^+$ helper T-cell phenotype. There are rare cases, however, of otherwise classical MF with a CD8$^+$/CD4$^-$/TIA1$^+$ immunophenotype that have the same clinical prognosis as conventional CD4$^+$ MF.[17] A T-cell clone can be identified in between 57% and 70% of cases of early patch-stage MF.[18,19]

The literature regarding loss of pan–T-cell antigens, such as CD2, CD5, and CD7, as assessed by immunohistochemistry, in the diagnosis of early MF has been discordant, with some studies

Fig. 15. MF, early patch stage. Subtle foci of epidermotropism of lesional lymphocytes. (HE, original magnification ×600).

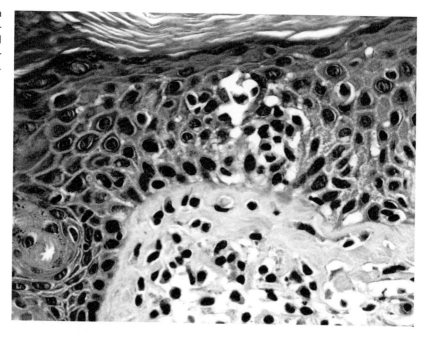

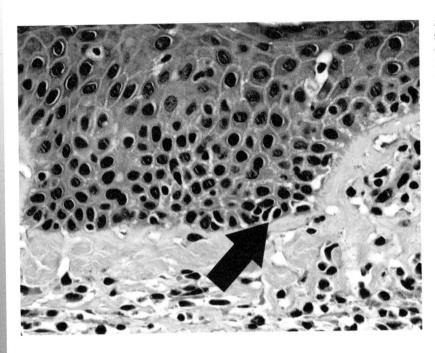

Fig. 16. MF, early patch stage. Subtle foci of epidermotropism of lesional lymphocytes (*arrow*) (HE, original magnification ×100).

demonstrating utility[20,21] and others showing nearly equal rates of loss in benign dermatoses.[14,22,23] One major difference between some of these studies are the benign dermatoses tested, because a study that showed usefulness of CD7 loss only used lichen planus, which is not usually a histopathologic mimic of MF, whereas a study demonstrating lack of specificity of CD7 loss used a group of controls that included psoriasis and spongiotic dermatitis, both of which can be difficult to distinguish from early MF, rendering it a more robust study.[14] It seems that loss of multiple T-cell markers within an epidermotropic infiltrate or discordant epidermal/dermal expression

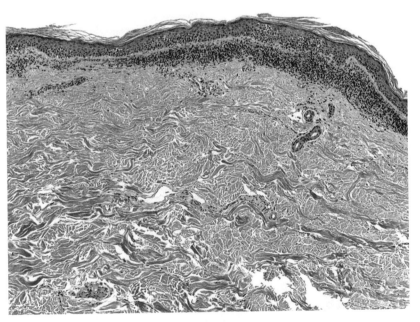

Fig. 17. MF, patch stage. Bandlike lymphocytic infiltrate within the papillary dermis with foci of epidermotropism of lymphocytes (HE, original magnification ×40).

Fig. 18. MF, patch stage. Well-developed foci of lymphocytes within the epidermis in the absence of spongiosis. (HE, original magnification ×400).

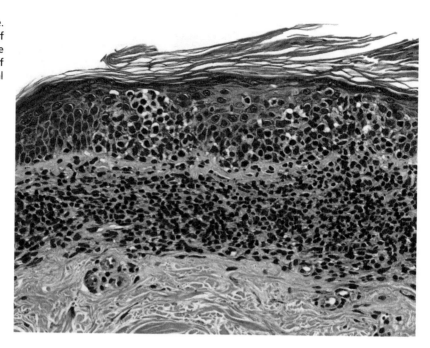

is relatively specific for MF, but these phenomena rarely occur in early disease.[24] Based on these data, and in this author's view, immunohistochemistry is rarely useful in diagnosing early MF.

The utility of detecting a T-cell clone using polymerase chain reaction (PCR)-based techniques in distinguishing early MF from histopathologic mimics has also been reported inconsistently in the literature. Some studies have demonstrated that a T-cell clone can be found in inflammatory dermatoses and can mimic early MF[25–28] whereas other studies have demonstrated very low rates of

Fig. 19. MF, patch stage. Foci of lymphocytes within the epidermis with minimal spongiosis (HE, original magnification ×200).

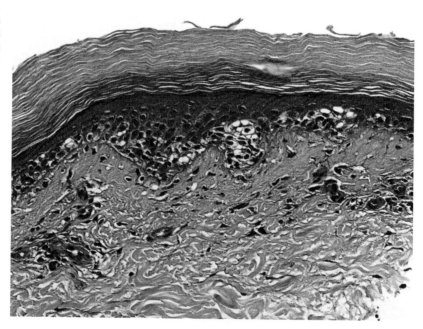

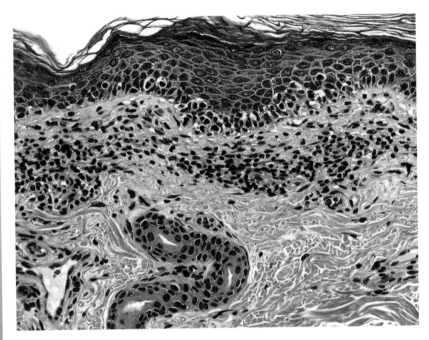

Fig. 20. MF, patch stage. Lymphocytes aligned along the basal layer of the epidermis (HE, original magnification ×200).

T-cell clone detection with inflammatory dermatoses.[18] Nonetheless, detection of the same clone from 2 anatomically distinct sites (also called dual T-cell receptor-PCR) seems to increase the sensitivity and specificity of T-cell clonality testing in diagnosing early MF.[29]

Due to the difficulty in rendering a definitive diagnosis of early MF, some authorities have advocated a scoring system with points awarded for clinical, histopathologic, immunophenotypic, and molecular data.[30] However, application of this algorithm to a group of

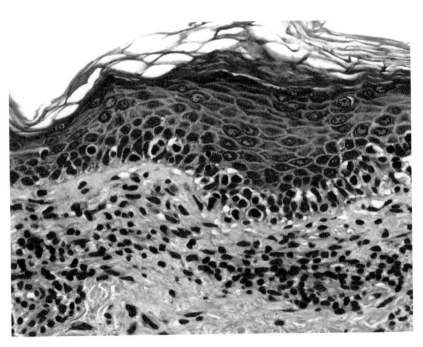

Fig. 21. MF, patch stage. Lymphocytes aligned along the basal layer of the epidermis. (HE, original magnification ×400).

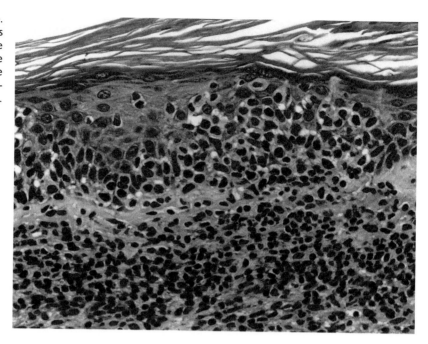

Fig. 22. MF, patch stage. The atypical lymphocytes within the epidermis are hyperchromatic and are slightly larger than those in the dermis (HE, original magnification ×600).

indeterminate cases demonstrated that ancillary testing generally was not helpful in further suggesting a diagnosis of MF when a definitive diagnosis could not be rendered.[31] Rather, an additional biopsy was the most helpful additional tool to render a definitive diagnosis in indeterminate cases, which has been the experience of this author as well.[31]

DIFFERENTIAL DIAGNOSIS

It can be challenging to distinguish early patch-stage MF, which frequently lacks atypical lymphocytes and is characterized by subtle epidermotropism, from inflammatory skin conditions, such as spongiotic dermatitis, psoriasis, a

Fig. 23. MF, plaque stage. Dense bandlike infiltrate of atypical lymphocytes extending into the upper reticular dermis. Intraepidermal collections of lymphocytes, also referred to as Pautrier microabscesses, are present (HE, original magnification ×100).

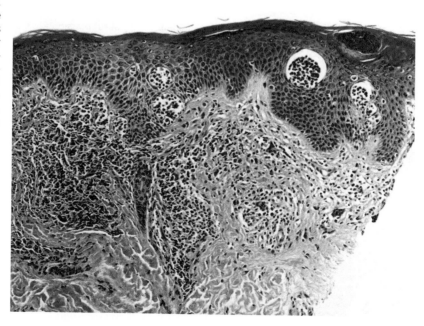

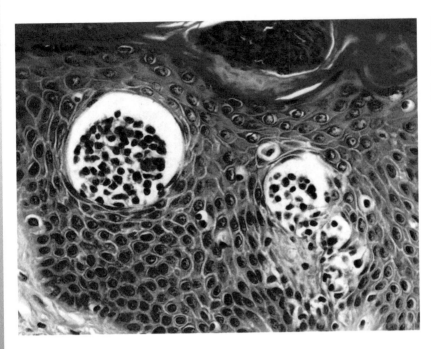

Fig. 24. MF, plaque stage. Detail view showing intraepidermal collections of atypical lymphocytes within the epidermis (HE, original magnification ×400).

dermatophytic (tinea) infection, a lymphomatoid drug reaction, lymphomatoid contact dermatitis, and chronic actinic dermatitis. In spongiotic dermatitis, intraepidermal collections of Langerhans cells frequently occur, which show some resemblance to the Pautrier collections seen in MF (**Figs. 34** and **35**), and it may be challenging to determine the cell type within the collections.

In such cases, immunohistochemistry with CD3 and CD1a can be helpful because these stains label T lymphocytes and Langerhans cells, respectively. Another difference is that collections of Langerhans cell tend to assume a vaselike shape, whereas Pautrier collections tend to be rounded (see **Fig. 35**).[32] Nonetheless, a sizable minority of early MF cases have been reported to demonstrate

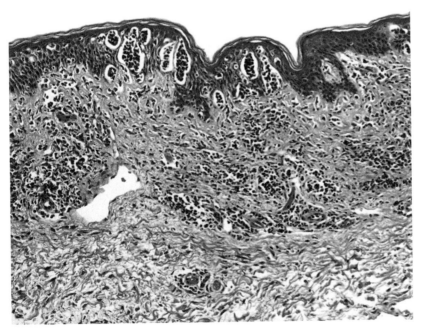

Fig. 25. MF, plaque stage. Numerous intraepidermal collections of neoplastic lymphocytes within the epidermis (HE, original magnification ×100).

Fig. 26. MF, plaque stage. Detailed view showing numerous intraepidermal collections of neoplastic lymphocytes within the epidermis (HE, original magnification ×400).

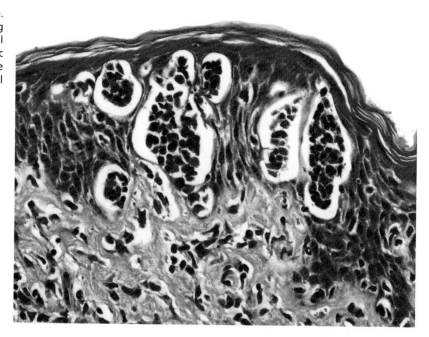

some degree of spongiosis,[12] making it difficult to distinguish spongiotic dermatitis from early MF. Psoriasis is distinguished from MF by the presence of dilated vessels in the dermal papillae, parakeratosis that contains neutrophils, and lack of epidermotropism. Dermatophytic infections lack epidermotropism as well, and there are periodic acid–Schiff (PAS)-positive hyphae in the stratum corneum. In lymphomatoid drug reactions and lymphomatoid allergic contact dermatitis, clinical follow-up is often necessary to differentiate from MF, because these eruptions tend to resolve after cessation of the causative medication or withdrawal of the contactant, respectively, although

Fig. 27. MF, plaque stage. Neoplastic lymphocytes within the upper dermis are somewhat atypical (HE, original magnification ×400).

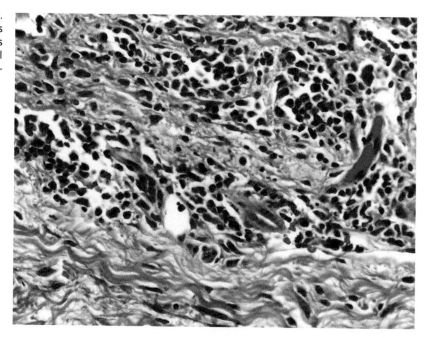

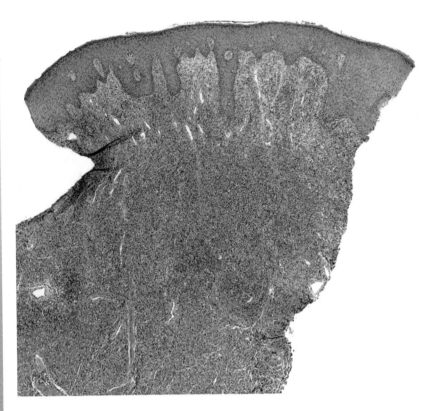

Fig. 28. MF, tumor stage. Dense and diffuse infiltrate involving the entire dermis composed of atypical lymphocytes (HE, original magnification ×40).

both conditions typically lack prominent epidermotropism.[33] Chronic actinic dermatitis often starts with lesions on photoexposed sites, and, when severe, may cause erythroderma. In general, the clinical presentation can be helpful in differentiating chronic actinic dermatitis from MF.

Other forms of lymphoma may show nearly identical histopathologic features to those seen

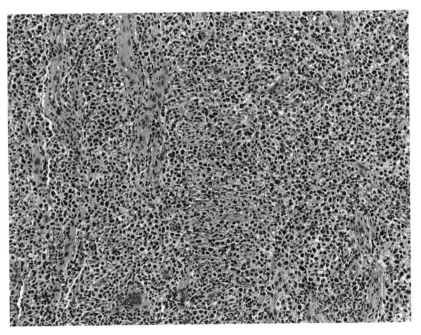

Fig. 29. MF, tumor stage. Neoplastic lymphocytes often form dense sheets in the dermis, illustrated here (HE, original magnification ×400).

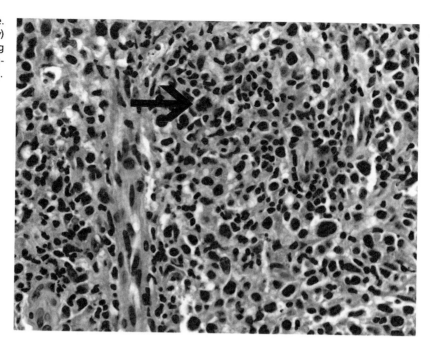

Fig. 30. MF, tumor stage. Mitotic figures (*arrow*) are often present among the lesional cells (HE, original magnification ×600).

in MF, including pagetoid reticulosis, types B and D lymphomatoid papulosis (LyP), primary cutaneous aggressive epidermotropic CD8⁺ T-cell lymphoma, Sézary syndrome, and adult T-cell leukemia/lymphoma (ATLL). The clinical presentation is required to distinguish between these types of lymphomas. In particular, pagetoid reticulosis presents as a solitary plaque on the distal

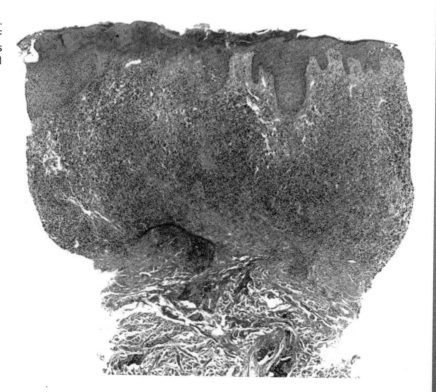

Fig. 31. MF, tumor stage. A case of tumor stage MF in which the epidermis is ulcerated (HE, original magnification ×40).

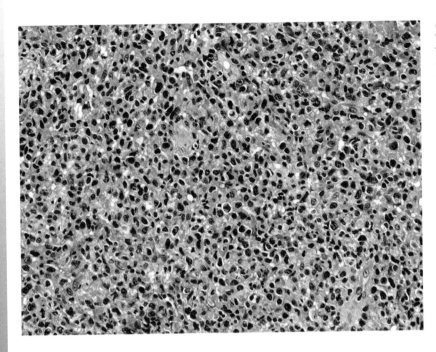

Fig. 32. MF, tumor stage with large cell transformation. Greater than 25% of the neoplastic lymphocytes are large (HE, original magnification ×200).

extremities; types B and D LyP typically with multiple recurring and self-healing papules and nodules; primary cutaneous aggressive epidermotropic CD8⁺ T-cell lymphoma with the sudden onset of multiple, often ulcerated plaques, and tumors without a history of long-standing patches and plaques; and Sézary syndrome with the sudden onset of erythroderma. ATLL can be histopathologically and clinically identical to MF, although ATLL is associated with clonal integration of the human T-lymphotropic virus (HTLV)-1 retrovirus, which MF is not.

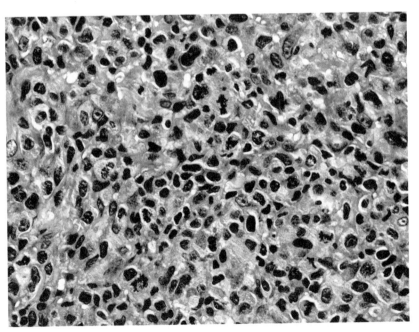

Fig. 33. MF, tumor stage with large cell transformation. Detailed view demonstrating that the majority of the neoplastic lymphocytes are large and that numerous mitotic figures are present (HE, original magnification ×600).

Fig. 34. Spongiotic dermatitis. Widening of the spaces between keratinocytes by intercellular edema (spongiosis) with collections of Langerhans cells in the epidermis (HE, original magnification ×400).

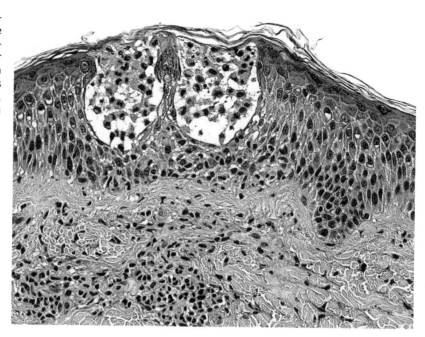

With regard to tumor-stage MF, other forms of lymphoma can show identical histopathologic findings, including primary cutaneous CD4+ small/medium pleomorphic T-cell lymphoma, anaplastic large cell lymphoma (ALCL), and LyP type C. In such cases, knowledge of the clinical presentation is necessary to formulate a specific diagnosis. In particular, primary cutaneous CD4+ small/medium pleomorphic T-cell lymphoma presents as a solitary papule or nodule, often on the upper body, with absence of patches/plaques elsewhere; ALCL is characterized by a solitary large ulcerated nodule; and LyP type C presents with multiple recurring and self-healing papules and nodules.

Fig. 35. Spongiotic dermatitis. High magnification of Langerhans cell collections with a vaselike configuration, in which the surface of the vase is present at the interface between the granular and cornified layers of the epidermis (HE, original magnification ×600).

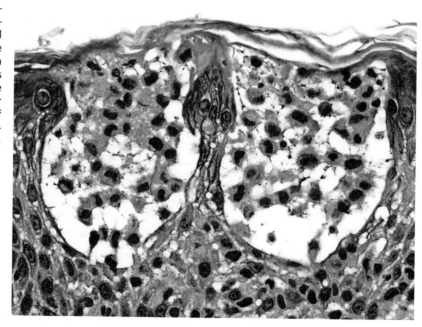

In summary, the diagnosis of all stages of MF rests on a clinical pathologic correlation, because there are many histopathologic mimics that can only be distinguished from MF by the clinical presentation. In its early stages, MF can be challenging to diagnose, and patients frequently are misdiagnosed with inflammatory forms of skin disease for years before receiving the correct diagnosis.[2] Due to the difficulty in establishing a definitive diagnosis of early patch-stage MF, repeat biopsies over time and ancillary studies, such as T-cell clonality testing, may prove helpful. Plaque-stage MF is typically easier to diagnose than patch-stage disease, because the infiltrate is usually denser and the epidermotropism often more pronounced. Knowledge of the clinical presentation is crucial, however, because patients should have concomitant patches. Similarly, a definitive diagnosis of tumor-stage MF should be established only if there is knowledge that the patient has concomitant patches and plaques of MF.

ΔΔ

Differential Diagnosis
PATCH/PLAQUE-STAGE MF

Mycosis Fungoides vs	Helpful Distinguishing Features
Spongiotic dermatitis	• Widened spaces between keratinocytes (spongiosis)
	• Lack of epidermotropism
	• Intraepidermal Langerhans cell collections assume a vaselike configuration and are CD1a$^+$/CD3$^-$
Psoriasis	• Parakeratosis that contains neutrophils
	• Lack of epidermotropism
Dermatophytic infection (tinea)	• Lack of epidermotropism
	• PAS-positive hyphae in cornified layer
Lymphomatoid drug eruption	• Lack of prominent epidermotropism
	• Clinical follow-up documenting resolution of the eruption with cessation of the medication
Lymphomatoid contact dermatitis	• Lack of prominent epidermotropism
	• Clinical follow-up documenting resolution of the eruption with withdrawal of the contactant
Chronic actinic dermatitis	• Lack of prominent epidermotropism
	• Involvement of photo-exposed sites in early-stage disease and erythroderma in end-stage disease[a]
Pagetoid reticulosis	• Clinically presents as a solitary patch or plaque on the distal extremities[a]
Types B and D LyP	• Clinically present as multiple recurring and self-healing papules and small nodules[a]
Primary cutaneous aggressive epidermotropic CD8$^+$ T-cell lymphoma	• Clinically presents the sudden onset of multiple, often ulcerated plaques and tumors[a]
Sézary syndrome	• Clinically presents with the sudden onset of erythroderma, along with lymphadenopathy and leukemic cells in the blood[a]
ATLL	• In patients from Japan or the Caribbean Islands
	• Clonal integration of the HTLV-1 retrovirus

[a] In contrast with MF, which typically presents with multiple large patches on photo-protected sites. In patients with disease progression, plaques and tumors develop, which are usually contiguous with preexisting patches.

Differential Diagnosis TUMOR-STAGE MF	
Mycosis Fungoides vs	**Helpful Distinguishing Features**
Primary cutaneous CD4$^+$ small/medium pleomorphic T-cell lymphoma	Solitary papule or nodule, often on the upper body[a]
Cutaneous ALCL	Solitary large ulcerated nodule[a]
Type C LyP	Multiple recurring and self-healing papules and small nodules[a]

[a] In contrast with MF, which typically presents with multiple large patches on photo-protected sites. In patients with disease progression, plaques and tumors develop, which are usually contiguous with preexisting patches.

PROGNOSIS

Prognosis varies by stage of disease, and all studies have demonstrated poorer survival with advancing stage of disease. Patients who die from MF typically either have systemic involvement or fatal infections.[1]

For patch/plaque-stage disease covering less than 10% body surface area (T1 disease/IA disease), 5- and 10-year disease-specific survival rates have been reported at 100% and 97%, respectively.[3] Relative survival rates compared with age-, gender-, and race-matched controls for T1 disease have been reported at 102.7% and 100.1 at 5 and 10 years, respectively.[34] This study demonstrated that T1 patients seem to have better survival compared with the control group composed of the general population.

For patch/plaque-stage disease covering greater than 10% body surface area (T2 disease/IB disease), disease-specific survival rates at 5 and 10 years have been reported at 96% and 83%, respectively,[3] whereas relative survival rates have been reported at 83.8% and 67.4%, respectively.[34]

In patients with tumors, 5- and 10-year disease-specific survival rates have been reported at 80% and 42%, respectively,[3] whereas relative 5- and 10-year survival rates have been reported at 51.5% and 39.8%, respectively.[34] For those patients who have developed erythroderma in the course of their disease, the relative 5- and 10-year survival rates have been reported at 57.3% and 41%, respectively.[34] When lymph nodes are involved, the 5- and 10-year disease-specific survival rates have been reported at 40% and 20%, respectively.[3] For those patients with visceral involvement, the 5- and 10-year disease-specific survival rates have been reported at 0% and 0%.[3]

The risk of disease progression seems to increase with advanced T classification. In particular, for T1 disease, the risk of disease progression at 5 and 10 years has been reported at 10% and 13%, respectively; for T2 disease, 22% and 32%, respectively; for T3 disease, 56% and 72%, respectively; and for T4 disease, 48% and 57%, respectively.[2]

Pitfalls
MYCOSIS FUNGOIDES

! Benign dermatoses, such as lymphomatoid allergic contact dermatitis and a lymphomatoid drug eruption, can histopathologically mimic patch/plaque-stage MF. Clinical correlation is needed to distinguish these entities.

! Many forms of cutaneous lymphoma can mimic MF. Therefore, a diagnosis of MF can only be rendered if the clinical presentation is compatible with the diagnosis.

! A CD8$^+$ immunophenotype in otherwise classical MF is not associated with a worse prognosis compared with a conventional CD4$^+$ immunophenotype.

! Assessment of T-cell immunophenotype is rarely helpful in the diagnosis of early MF.

! Although the detection of a T-cell clone favors MF, it is not pathognomonic for MF, because T-cell clones can occasionally be detected in benign dermatoses.

REFERENCES

1. Willemze R, Jaffe ES, Burg G, et al. WHO-EORTC classification for cutaneous lymphomas. Blood 2005;105: 3768–85.
2. Kim YH, Liu HL, Mraz-Gernhard S, et al. Long-term outcome of 525 patients with mycosis fungoides and Sézary syndrome: clinical prognostic factors and risk for disease progression. Arch Dermatol 2003;139:857–66.
3. van Doorn R, Van Haselen CW, van Voorst Vader PC, et al. Mycosis fungoides: disease evolution and prognosis of 309 Dutch patients. Arch Dermatol 2000;136:504–10.
4. Weinstock MA, Gardstein B. Twenty-year trends in the reported incidence of mycosis fungoides and associated mortality. Am J Public Health 1999;89: 1240–4.
5. Criscione VD, Weinstock MA. Incidence of cutaneous T-cell lymphoma in the United States, 1973-2002. Arch Dermatol 2007;143:854–9.
6. Weinstock MA, Horm JW. Mycosis fungoides in the United States. Increasing incidence and descriptive epidemiology. JAMA 1988;260:42–6.
7. Olsen E, Vonderheid E, Pimpinelli N, et al. Revisions to the staging and classification of mycosis fungoides and Sézary syndrome: a proposal of the International Society for Cutaneous Lymphomas (ISCL) and the cutaneous lymphoma task force of the European Organization of Research and Treatment of Cancer (EORTC). Blood 2007; 110:1713–22.
8. Zackheim HS, McCalmont TH, Deanovic FW, et al. Mycosis fungoides with onset before 20 years of age. J Am Acad Dermatol 1997;36:557–62.
9. Sanchez JL, Ackerman AB. The patch stage of mycosis fungoides. Criteria for histologic diagnosis. Am J Dermatopathol 1979;1:5–26.
10. Massone C, Kodama K, Kerl H, et al. Histopathologic features of early (patch) lesions of mycosis fungoides: a morphologic study on 745 biopsy specimens from 427 patients. Am J Surg Pathol 2005;29:550–60.
11. Gellrich S, Lukowsky A, Schilling T, et al. Microanatomical compartments of clonal and reactive T cells in mycosis fungoides: molecular demonstration by single cell polymerase chain reaction of T cell receptor gene rearrangements. J Invest Dermatol 2000; 115:620–4.
12. Nickoloff BJ. Light-microscopic assessment of 100 patients with patch/plaque-stage mycosis fungoides. Am J Dermatopathol 1988;10:469–77.
13. LeBoit PE, McCalmont TH. Cutaneous lymphomas and leukemias. In: Elder D, editor. Lever's histopathology of the skin. 8th edition. Philadelphia: Lippincott–Raven Publishers; 1997. p. 805–46.
14. Florell SR, Cessna M, Lundell RB, et al. Usefulness (or lack thereof) of immunophenotyping in atypical cutaneous T-cell infiltrates. Am J Clin Pathol 2006; 125:727–36.
15. Salhany KE, Cousar JB, Greer JP, et al. Transformation of cutaneous T cell lymphoma to large cell lymphoma. A clinicopathologic and immunologic study. Am J Pathol 1988;132:265–77.
16. Vergier B, de Muret A, Beylot-Barry M, et al. Transformation of mycosis fungoides: clinicopathological and prognostic features of 45 cases. Blood 2000; 95:2212–8.
17. Massone C, Crisman G, Kerl H, et al. The prognosis of early mycosis fungoides is not influenced by phenotype and T-cell clonality. Br J Dermatol 2008; 159:881–6.
18. Ponti R, Quaglino P, Novelli M, et al. T-cell receptor gamma gene rearrangement by multiplex polymerase chain reaction/heteroduplex analysis in patients with cutaneous T-cell lymphoma (mycosis fungoides/Sézary syndrome) and benign inflammatory disease: correlation with clinical, histological and immunophenotypical findings. Br J Dermatol 2005; 153:565–73.
19. Bachelez H, Bioul L, Flageul B, et al. Detection of clonal T-cell receptor gamma gene rearrangements with the use of the polymerase chain reaction in cutaneous lesions of mycosis fungoides and Sézary syndrome. Arch Dermatol 1995;131: 1027–31.
20. Ormsby A, Bergfeld WF, Tubbs RR, et al. Evaluation of a new paraffin-reactive CD7 T-cell deletion marker and a polymerase chain reaction-based T-cell receptor gene rearrangement assay: implications for diagnosis of mycosis fungoides in community clinical practice. J Am Acad Dermatol 2001;45:405–13.
21. Bergman R, Faclieru D, Sahar D, et al. Immunophenotyping and T-cell receptor gamma gene rearrangement analysis as an adjunct to the histopathologic diagnosis of mycosis fungoides. J Am Acad Dermatol 1998;39:554–9.
22. Stevens SR, Ke MS, Birol A, et al. A simple clinical scoring system to improve the sensitivity and standardization of the diagnosis of mycosis fungoides type cutaneous T-cell lymphoma: logistic regression of clinical and laboratory data. Br J Dermatol 2003; 149:513–22.
23. Ralfkiaer E, Wantzin GL, Mason DY, et al. Phenotypic characterization of lymphocyte subsets in mycosis fungoides. Comparison with large plaque parapsoriasis and benign chronic dermatoses. Am J Clin Pathol 1985;84:610–9.
24. Michie SA, Abel EA, Hoppe RT, et al. Discordant expression of antigens between intraepidermal and intradermal T cells in mycosis fungoides. Am J Pathol 1990;137:1447–51.

25. Schiller PI, Flaig MJ, Puchta U, et al. Detection of clonal T cells in lichen planus. Arch Dermatol Res 2000;292:568–9.

26. Dereure O, Levi E, Kadin ME. T-cell clonality in pityriasis lichenoides et varioliformis acuta. Arch Dermatol 2000;136:1483–6.

27. Shieh S, Mikkola DL, Wood GS. Differentiation and clonality of lesional lymphocytes in pityriasis lichenoides chronica. Arch Dermatol 2001;137:305–8.

28. Lukowsky A, Muche JM, Sterry W, et al. Detection of expanded T cell clones in skin biopsy samples of patients with lichen sclerosus et atrophicus by T cell receptor-g polymerase chain reaction assays. J Invest Dermatol 2000;115:254–9.

29. Thurber SE, Zhang B, Kim YH, et al. T-cell clonality analysis in biopsy specimens from two different skin sites shows high specificity in the diagnosis of patients with suggested mycosis fungoides. J Am Acad Dermatol 2007;57:782–90.

30. Pimpinelli N, Olsen EA, Santucci M, et al. Defining early mycosis fungoides. J Am Acad Dermatol 2005;53:1053–63.

31. Ferrara G, Di Blasi A, Zalaudek I, et al. Regarding the algorithm for the diagnosis of early mycosis fungoides proposed by the International Society for Cutaneous Lymphomas: suggestions from routine histopathology practice. J Cutan Pathol 2008;35:549–53.

32. LeBoit PE, Epstein BA. A vase-like shape characterizes the epidermal-mononuclear cell collections seen in spongiotic dermatitis. Am J Dermatopathol 1990;12:612–6.

33. Rijlaarsdam JU, Scheffer E, Meijer CJ, et al. Cutaneous pseudo-T-cell lymphomas. A clinicopathologic study of 20 patients. Cancer 1992;69:717–24.

34. Zackheim HS, Amin S, Kashani-Sabet M, et al. Prognosis in cutaneous T-cell lymphoma by skin stage: long-term survival in 489 patients. J Am Acad Dermatol 1999;40:418–25.

Mycosis Fungoides Variants

M. Estela Martínez-Escala, MD[a,b], Belén Rubio González, MD[c], Joan Guitart, MD[a,b,d],*

KEYWORDS

- Clinicopathologic variants • Folliculotropic mycosis fungoides • Granulomatous slack skin
- Hypopigmented mycosis fungoides • Pagetoid reticulosis • Woringer-Kolopp disease

KEY POINTS

- Mycosis fungoides (MF) is the most common subtype of cutaneous T-cell lymphoma (CTCL), and its diagnosis is often challenging for clinicians and the pathologists. The early clinical stages may resemble an inflammatory process, and a significant component of the lymphoid infiltrate may be reactive rather than neoplastic.
- Proper correlation between clinical features, pathologic findings, and molecular and immunohistochemical analysis is essential to reach the correct diagnosis.
- In particular, MF variants may be difficult to diagnose. Clinicians and pathologists should be aware of these important MF variants, because their diagnosis is frequently delayed or misdiagnosed.

ABSTRACT

Mycosis fungoides (MF) is a cutaneous T-cell lymphoma that usually manifests as patches and plaques with a propensity for nonphotoexposed areas. MF is a common mimicker of inflammatory and infectious skin diseases, because it can be manifested with a wide variety of clinical and pathologic presentations. These atypical presentations of MF may be difficult to diagnose, requiring a high level of suspicion and careful clinicopathologic correlation. Within this array of clinical presentations, the World Health Organization classification recognizes 3 MF variants: folliculotropic MF, pagetoid reticulosis, and granulomatous slack skin. These 3 variants, as well as hypopigmented MF, are addressed in this article.

OVERVIEW

MF is the most common CTCL, clinically manifested with scaly erythematous patches that may evolve to plaques and tumor lesions. Histologically, a superficial bandlike infiltrate of small and medium-sized atypical T cells tends to be associated with epidermotropism and reticular fibroplasia of the papillary dermis. The most common phenotype of the neoplastic cells are CD2$^+$, CD3$^+$, CD5$^+$, CD4$^+$, CD7$^-$, CD8$^-$, CD45RO$^+$, T-cell receptor (TCR) β$^+$, and CD30$^-$.[1] But deletion of several pan–T-cell markers may also be observed. Besides the classical features of MF, first described by Alibert in 1806, there are many variable clinical and histopathologic presentations that differ substantially from the classical or conventional presentation and that can mimic a variety of inflammatory skin diseases.[2,3] Practically all patterns of inflammatory dermatoses have been described in patients with MF. Thus, a diagnosis of MF can become highly challenging to dermatologists and pathologists alike.

Clinicopathologic presentations other than the conventional MF presentation include[1] folliculotropic, syringotropic, erythrodermic, granulomatous, poikilodermic, lichenoid, hypopigmented,

Disclosure Statement: The authors declare no financial disclosure.
[a] Department of Dermatology, Feinberg School of Medicine, Northwestern University, 676 North Saint Clair Street, Suite 1600, Chicago, IL 60611, USA; [b] Department of Pathology, Feinberg School of Medicine, Northwestern University, 676 North Saint Clair Street, Suite 1600, Chicago, IL 60611, USA; [c] Dermatology Department, Hospital 12 de Octubre, Avda de Córdoba s/n, 28041 - Madrid, Spain; [d] Division of Hematology/Oncology Department, Robert H. Lurie Comprehensive Cancer Center, 675 North Saint Clair Street, Suite 19 100, Chicago, IL 60611, USA
* Corresponding author. Department of Dermatology, Feinberg School of Medicine, Northwestern University, 676 North Saint Clair Street, Suite 1600, Chicago, IL 60611.
E-mail address: j-guitart@northwestern.edu

Surgical Pathology 7 (2014) 169–189
http://dx.doi.org/10.1016/j.path.2014.02.003
1875-9181/14/$ – see front matter © 2014 Elsevier Inc. All rights reserved.

surgpath.theclinics.com

hyperpigmented, pagetoid reticulosis (PR), pigmented purpura-like, bullous/vesicular, palmoplantar, hyperkeratotic/verrucous, vegetating/papillomatous, ichthyosiform, interstitial, papular, and invisible.

The latest World Health Organization (WHO) classification of cutaneous lymphomas officially recognizes only 3 MF variants as entities with different presentation, clinical behavior, and treatment response compared with classical MF.[4] These variants include folliculotropic MF (FMF), PR (localized Woringer-Kolopp type), and granulomatous slack skin syndrome (GSSS).[4] This article focuses on these 3 subtypes, along with hypopigmented MF (HMF), and briefly mentions other unusual rare variants.

FOLLICULOTROPIC MYCOSIS FUNGOIDES

OVERVIEW

The T lymphocytes in FMF have a peculiar tropism for follicular epithelium. This fairly common presentation of MF has been recognized since the early 1960s. The mechanism attracting neoplastic T cells to follicular units is not known. It is hypothesized that high density of antigen-presenting cells (CD1a$^+$ Langerhans cells) within follicular epithelia may lead to localized chronic antigenic stimulation to T cells as a precursor process.[5,6] An alternative explanation is that FMF arises from distinct T-cell subsets with homing to the pilosebaceous unit. To that effect, a gene expression study showed

Key Histologic Features OF FOLLICULOTROPIC MYCOSIS FUNGOIDES

Main feature: atypical lymphocytic infiltrate mostly localized in pilosebaceous units

Five patterns (concomitant or as a sole feature):

1. Mucinous deposits in the follicular unit

2. Granulomatous reaction with destruction of follicular epithelium

3. Eosinophilic folliculitis–like presentation

4. Cystic and comedonal changes

5. Basaloid folliculolymphoid hyperplasia with folliculotropism

Immunophenotype

- CD3$^+$, CD4$^+$, CD7$^-$

- Abundant CD1a cells in follicular epithelia

prevalence of specific pathways involved in inflammation and benign epidermal hyperproliferation in most of the FMF analyzed.[7] The WHO classification of cutaneous lymphomas recognizes FMF as a distinct entity, due to its unique clinical and histopathologic features, survival outcome, and therapeutic responses compared with classical MF.[4,8]

CLINICAL FEATURES

FMF are typically manifested on skin sites rich in pilosebaceous units, such as head, neck, and upper torso. The presence of erythematous scaly patches and plaques with follicular-based papules associated with intense pruritus is the most frequent clinical presentation (**Fig. 1A**).[9] The areas of involvement differ from conventional MF by an ill-defined appearance, frequent hair loss, and distinct distribution of the lesions. Generalized erythroderma at the initial presentation is rarely observed. The authors have observed that FMF can resemble the entire spectrum of pathologic conditions involving the pilosebaceous unit, including a wide array of alopecias and acneiform presentations. The spectrum of mimicked conditions observed includes inflammatory acneiform lesions, acne conglobata, comedone, cysts, milia (milia en plaques), lichen spinulosus, keratosis pilaris–like papules on the legs and arm, and alopecia that can resemble alopecia areata, lichen planopilaris, trichotillomania, and folliculitis decalvans (see **Fig. 1B–D**; **Fig. 2**). Due to intense pruritus, patients tend to scratch the lesions and may develop excoriated papules with crust formation and impetiginized erosions, giving rise to prurigo nodularis–like lesions that can resemble tumor progression.[5,6,8,10] Rarely, patients may exhibit mucinorrhoea (discharge of mucinous substance from follicular orifices), which is highly characteristic of this entity and is usually associated with follicular mucinosis as a histopathologic finding. Nodal and peripheral blood involvement is rarely identified, at least in the early stages.[9] FMF has significantly higher male-to-female ratio (4–5: 1) compared with conventional MF, and it has been reported that women have an older age of onset than in men.[9] Rare cases have been reported in children.[11]

DIAGNOSIS: MICROSCOPIC FEATURES

The infiltrate is mostly localized to the pilosebaceous unit, with fewer cases also showing epidermal involvement. Atypical lymphocytes can involve any of the components of the follicular unit and the infiltrate can result in mucinous

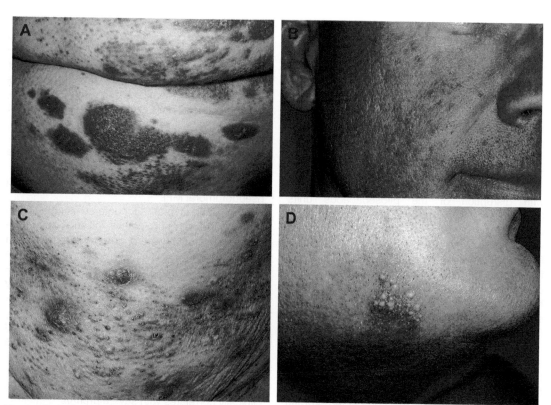

Fig. 1. Clinical manifestations of FMF. (*A*) Erythematous follicular-based and confluent plaques on the trunk. (*B*) Acnelike presentation. (*C*) Confluent comedones with erythematous nodules on the lower abdomen. (*D*) Erythematous plaque with milia on the right jaw.

degeneration or in some cases complete disruption and necrosis of the follicular epithelium with secondary suppurative or granulomatous inflammation. Syringotropism to the eccrine sweat glands can also be present, even as a sole feature if the biopsy lacks follicular structures for examination. Due to the wide variety of clinical

manifestations, it is not surprising that FMF may also manifest with a variety of histologic patterns. Five histologic patterns are described[5,6]: (1) the prototypical folliculotropic infiltrate of atypical lymphocytes with or without mucinous deposits; (2) granulomatous reaction: granulomatous dermatitis closely associated with a destructive process of

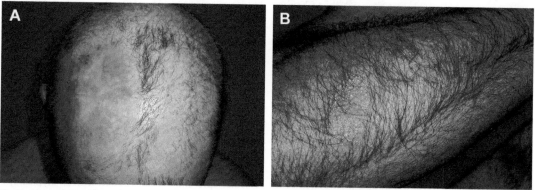

Fig. 2. Clinical manifestations of FMF. (*A*) Alopecia areata–like patches. (*B*) Alopecic patch with keratosis pilaris–like changes on the right arm.

the follicular unit with evidence of folliculotropism; (3) eosinophilic folliculitis–like presentation with folliculotropism; (4) cystic and comedonal changes: formation of dilated follicular cysts with folliculotropism; and (5) basaloid folliculolymphoid hyperplasia with folliculotropism. Multiple biopsies may reveal different patterns and even different patterns can be observed within a single biopsy specimen.[8]

The folliculotropic infiltrate of atypical lymphocytes is the most frequently recognized pattern. The second granulomatous pattern is associated with disruption of the pilosebaceous units (Fig. 3A). The granulomatous changes are observed directly adjacent to a follicle distended with mucin and lymphocytes or infundibular cyst formation with keratin retention (see Fig. 3B). These findings are commonly associated with prototypical folliculotropic infiltrate (first pattern), which helps reach a diagnosis. The third pattern describes eosinophilic folliculitis–like changes, frequently detected as a sole finding, with the atypical lymphocytes overshadowed by the amount of eosinophils, which makes the diagnosis difficult (see Fig. 3A). Follicular cystic changes are characteristic in the fourth pattern, occasionally associated with accumulation of compacted keratin

(Fig. 4). Mucinous deposits are not constant, although large intrafollicular cystic pools may be observed. This histologic pattern is clinically correlated with acneiform lesions, comedones, or keratosis pilaris–like changes. The fifth pattern is uncommon and identified by basaloid proliferations of epithelial cells extending from either intact or completely transformed hair follicles (Fig. 5A). Mucinous deposition is frequent in this pattern. The follicular hyperplasia may clinically correlate with elevated lesions, resembling tumors of disease, without being true tumor lesions (so-called pseudotumoral MF).

Other findings rarely encountered include pustular changes with suppurative follicular inflammation, an interstitial and/or interface pattern with variable epidermotropism of nonfollicular epithelium (see Fig. 5B). Many biopsies also reveal histologic features associated with pruritus as noted by the presence of superficial excoriations, extravasation of erythrocytes, lamellar fibroplasia of the papillary dermis, acanthosis, focal spongiosis, and superimposed features of lichen simplex chronicus or prurigo nodularis. Unlike conventional MF, eosinophils and plasma cells are often conspicuous within the accompanying reactive infiltrate, which clinically correlates with severe pruritus.[8]

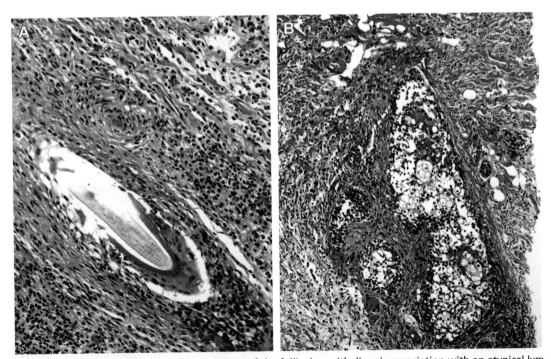

Fig. 3. Histologic features of FMF. (A) Destruction of the follicular epithelium in association with an atypical lymphocytic infiltrate with eosinophils (HE, original magnification ×40). (B) Mucinous disruption of follicular architecture accompanied with an atypical lymphocytic infiltrate (HE, original magnification ×20).

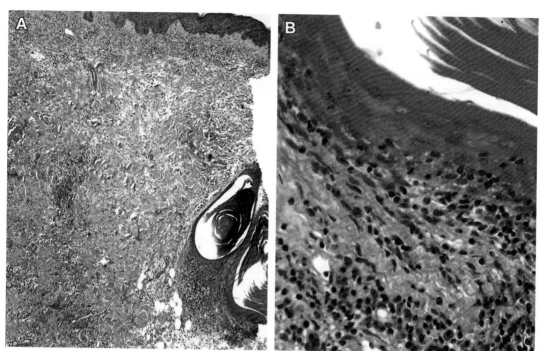

Fig. 4. Histologic features of FMF. (*A*) Perifollicular lymphocytic infiltrate with follicular cystic changes and accumulation of compacted keratin (HE, original magnification ×10). (*B*) High-power magnification showing the folliculotropic lymphocytic infiltrate (HE, original magnification ×40).

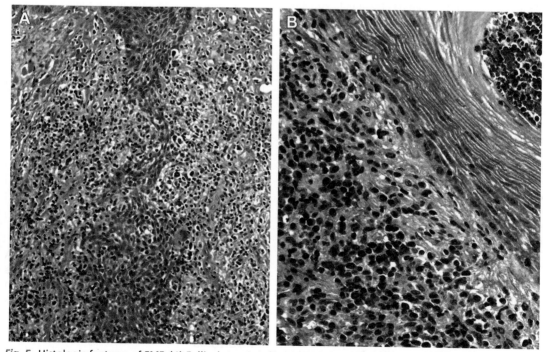

Fig. 5. Histologic features of FMF. (*A*) Folliculotropic infiltrate with basaloid features (HE, original magnification ×20). (*B*) Atypical perifollicular infiltrate and nuclear debris in the lumen of the hair follicle (HE, original magnification ×40).

DIAGNOSIS: ANCILLARY STUDIES

The immunophenotype of FMF does not differ from conventional MF, with $CD3^+$, $CD4^+$, $CD7^-$ cells and an overall CD4:CD8 ratio of the infiltrate that tends to be higher than 6:1. Follicular epithelia may show abundant $CD1a^+$ cells.[6,8] TCR gene rearrangement clonality is frequently (82%) detected.[8]

DIFFERENTIAL DIAGNOSIS

As previously discussed, FMF may clinically simulate a variety of alopecias and inflammatory conditions involving the follicular unit. Adult-onset comedocystic acne, papulopustular or granulomatous rosacea, chronic folliculitis, eosinophilic folliculitis, and even Favre-Racouchot syndrome and chloracne (due to exposure to halogenated aromatic compounds) may be considered in the differential diagnosis. The authors have also observed cases resembling alopecia areata, trichotillomania, and cicatricial alopecias. Unusual distribution of the lesions, follicular prominence, alopecia, and pruritus are clues that may help reach a diagnosis. Cases of coexisting FMF and other forms of inflammatory alopecias or folliculitis, however, have been reported.[6,8]

Idiopathic follicular mucinosis (IFM) represents one of the most difficult differential diagnoses both clinically and histologically.[1,12–14] IFM usually manifests as localized lesions and affects younger patients, in contrast with FMF.[12] Abundant mucin deposition within the hair follicles, sometimes leading to their destruction, and patchy lymphohistiocytic perifollicular infiltrates are the main histologic features. It is associated with a benign course, even though the course is protracted and tends to be recalcitrant to various therapies. Histologic differentiation between IFM and FMF can be difficult or even impossible when based on just one biopsy. Clinical follow-up and serial biopsies may be needed in some cases. Careful clinicopathologic correlation is mandatory to reach a proper diagnosis. Moreover, the relationship between IFM and MF remains controversial.[5,12–15] It has been suggested that IFM might be an indolent form of CTCL or a cutaneous T-cell lymphoid dyscrasia (CLD), with frequent T-cell clonality and even progression to bona fide MF reported in rare cases.[16,17]

Histologically, the granulomatous pattern sometimes observed in FMF may be confused with granulomatous MF, which in general should be considered a distinct, albeit not formally recognized, variant of CTCL, and is often associated with $CD8^+$ phenotype. This latter variant manifests as erythematous to violaceous nodules or plaques

> ## △△ Differential Diagnosis
> ## OF FOLLICULOTROPIC MYCOSIS FUNGOIDES
>
> A. Clinical
>   1. Acneiform conditions
>   - Adult-onset comedocystic acne
>   - Acne conglobata
>   - Rosacea: papulopustular or granulomatous
>   - Folliculitis: chronic, eosinophilic
>   - Favre-Racouchot syndrome
>   - Chloracne
>   2. Alopecia
>   - Alopecia areata
>   - Trichotillomania
>   - Cicatricial alopecias
>   3. Others
>   - Lichen spinulosus
>   - Keratosis pilaris
>   - IFM
>   - Leonine facies (leprosy)
> B. Histologic
>   1. Mucinous deposits in the follicular unit
>   - IFM
>   2. Granulomatous reaction with destruction of follicular unit
>   - $CD8^+$ granulomatous MF
>   - Large cell transformation of MF
>   - Tumor-stage MF
>   3. Eosinophilic folliculitis–like
>   - Eosinophilic folliculitis
>   4. Cystic and comedonal changes
>   - Favre-Racouchot syndrome
>   - Comedocystic acne

that lack follicular-based papules and alopecia. A clinical and pathologic diagnostic pitfall of this granulomatous presentation of FMF is that it can be misdiagnosed as tumor progression or large cell transformation of MF.

PROGNOSIS

Several studies have shown that FMF tends to be more recalcitrant and overall more aggressive than conventional MF.[5,9,18] Difficulties in achieving a good response with skin-directed therapies, even in early cases, may be related to the depth of the malignant infiltrate out of reach of skin-directed therapies, including UV-B. Thus, systemic agents are required in most cases to induce a remission. Psoralen plus UV-A (PUVA) therapy with oral bexarotene or acitretin and PUVA with interferon alfa have shown good outcomes. Total skin electron beam monotherapy or in combination with retinoids or interferon has also been demonstrated as effective and well tolerated, achieving persistent prolonged remissions.[17] Patients with more advanced disease (≥IIB) require more aggressive systemic therapy. Irradiation and allogeneic stem cell transplantation have shown better results compared with conventional chemotherapies, such as gemcitabine, liposomal doxorubicin, and cyclophosphamide, doxorubicin, vincristine, and prednisone (CHOP).

Pruritus is a common complaint with high impact on patient quality of life and treatment is difficult. Several therapeutic approaches have failed to control this clinical symptom, which is often aggravated by *Staphylococcus aureus* infection. Pruritus tends to improve with successful lymphoma treatment. Adjuvant therapies that may ameliorate pruritus include antihistamines and psychotropic drugs, such as doxepin, amitriptyline, pregabalin, and gabapentin. Topical therapies also include lowering the ambient temperature to decrease the triggering threshold, emollients, antibacterial soaks, antibiotics, and chlorine bleach baths to control bacterial colonization and superinfection.[5]

Overall FMF has shown an increase risk of disease progression. Marked differences in prognosis are observed between FMF and conventional MF, especially within the early disease stages (≤IIA). The overall survival of patients with stage IIA or lower was 82% for FMF and 91% for MF at 10 years, falling to 41% in FMF while remaining stable (91%) at 15 years in conventional MF.[5] This can be explained by the difficulty in achieving complete response in early-stage disease with the use of skin-directed therapies. Patients with advanced disease (IIB or higher) have similar poor outcome compared with conventional MF.

PAGETOID RETICULOSIS (WORINGER-KOLOPP DISEASE)

OVERVIEW

PR is a rare variant of MF formally recognized in the latest WHO classification. PR was first

Key Histologic Features
OF PAGETOID RETICULOSIS

Main feature: massive intraepidermal infiltrate of medium to large lymphocytes

Other features occasionally present:

- Verrucous or corrugated epidermis

- Serohemorrhagic crust or ulceration

Immunophenotype

- $CD3^+$, $CD4^+$, $CD8^-$; or $CD3^+$, $CD4^-$, $CD8^+$; or $CD3^+$, $CD4^-$, $CD8^-$

- $CD45RO^+$, $BF-1^+$

- $TIA-1^\pm$, $CD56^-$

- CD30 variable

described by Frederic Woringer and Pierre Kolopp in 1939, in a 13-year-old boy with a lesion on his forearm of 6 years of evolution. Since then, many cases have been reported, often in children and young adults.[19] The term PR should be exclusively used for patients with localized disease with a single or a few clustered lesions.[20,21] There has been some debate about the pathomechanistic nature of PR, whether Woringer-Kolopp disease is a true lymphoma or a benign lymphoproliferative process akin to lymphomatoid papulosis (LyP) that occasionally may evolve to MF.[22]

CLINICAL FEATURES

PR typically manifests as asymptomatic, slowly growing, hyperkeratotic, and often verrucous plaques localized preferable in acral areas, ranging in size from small papules of less than 1 cm to large plaques of more than 30 cm (**Fig. 6A**). Patients can present with a single lesion or with few lesions, which may become confluent, and involving the same anatomic regions, most commonly upper or lower extremities. Ulceration, often associated with pain, is observed in some cases. An exceptional case of a papule located on the tongue has been reported.[23] If the process is extensive, however, and especially if oral involvement is also noted, other variants of CTCL, such as primary cutaneous aggressive epidermotropic $CD8^+$ T-cell lymphoma ($CD8^+$ PCAETCL), commonly known as Berti lymphoma, should be suspected. Nodal or systemic involvement is typically absent.[4]

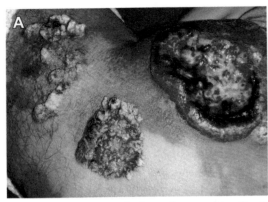
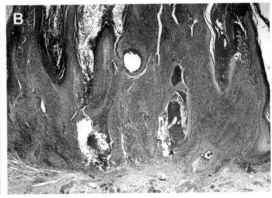

Fig. 6. Clinicopathologic findings of a case of localized PR. (*A*) Ulcerated tumor—plaque lesions with sharply well demarcated borders and variable hyperkeratotic changes. (*B*) Hyperkeratotic and verrucoid epidermal changes associated with dense lichenoid lymphocytic infiltrate in the papillary dermis (HE, original magnification ×4).

DIAGNOSIS: MICROSCOPIC FEATURES

The main histopathologic feature of PR is the massive intraepidermal infiltrate of medium- to large-sized lymphocytes, which occupies the entire thickness of the epidermis exhibiting a prominent pagetoid pattern. The infiltrate tends to be monomorphous, but some pleomorphism and hyperchromasia may be observed. Cerebriform nuclei similar to MF cells occasionally are observed.[21,24] A clear halo around the cell compressing the adjacent keratinocytes, often accompanied by some nuclear debris, also is commonly observed. Marked acanthosis and corrugation of the epidermis, in some cases resulting in verrucous hyperplasia, also are commonly noted (see **Fig. 6**B); the rapid growth and hyperplastic changes may result in erosive changes with serohemorrhagic crusting or, in some cases, frank ulceration.

DIAGNOSIS: ANCILLARY STUDIES

Three different immunophenotypes are described in PR: (1) CD4-positive T-helper phenotype (CD3$^+$, CD4$^+$, CD8$^-$); (2) T-cytotoxic/suppressor phenotype (CD3$^+$, CD4$^-$, CD8$^+$); and (3) double-negative phenotype (CD3$^+$, CD4$^-$, CD8$^-$). The T cells are mostly mature with positive CD45RO expression, although the authors have observed rare cases of expression of the naïve phenotype CD45RA$^+$, which is more typical of the generalized and aggressive CD8$^+$ PCAETCL. Expression of CD30 is variable, but it is often expressed in a majority of intraepidermal neoplastic cells. TCR-β (βF-1) is mostly positive, and T-cell intracytoplasmic antigen-1 (TIA-1) is positive in those cases of expression of CD8 or a null CD4$^-$/CD8$^-$ phenotype. CD56 is usually negative.[25] TCR gene rearrangement clonality may be detected.[4]

DIFFERENTIAL DIAGNOSIS

The clinical differential diagnosis of PR should include papulosquamous, neoplastic, and infectious conditions. PR can clinically manifest as a plaque of chronic eczema, psoriasiform dermatitis (hyperkeratotic plaques), or infectious conditions, such as tuberculosis verrucosa cutis, blastomycosis, leishmania, dermatophyte infection, or a verrucous process. Special stains for microorganisms and even tissue culture may be required when granulomatous or suppurative changes are noted, especially in erosive cases.

Certain cutaneous malignancies, including CD30$^+$ lymphoproliferative conditions, verrucous squamous cell carcinoma, and verrucous melanoma, may also be associated with pseudoepitheliomatous hyperplasia and should be considered in the differential diagnosis. Histology and immunohistochemistry studies help differentiate between these skin cancers.

Certain CTCL variants may be differentiated clinically and histologically from PR. PR manifested on thighs or buttocks areas can be confused with the so-called unilesional MF variant; however, the striking intraepidermal infiltrate seen in PR is absent in these cases. MF palmaris et plantaris, an extraordinary MF variant manifested with lesions limited to the palms and/or soles, may also be considered in the differential diagnosis. It has a high variety of manifestations, including annular and hyperpigmented patches and plaques, vesicles or dyshidrotic lesions, pustules, and ulceration, but often lesions are hyperkeratotic, verrucous, or psoriasiform plaques. Nail dystrophy may be present. Lesions are usually bilateral, a major distinction from PR, and palms are more frequently affected than soles.[26,27] The main differential diagnosis of MF palmaris et plantaris is with eczematous dermatitis, which in nonglabrous skin often presents with dense lymphoid infiltrate with marked exocytosis. This presentation may be confused with MF and PR. The authors have also observed extraordinary cases of CD30[+] lymphoproliferative disorders with eczematoid or hyperkeratotic plaques involving palms and soles.

Cases previously reported in the literature as the generalized form of PR, or Ketron-Goodman type, are now considered other CTCL variants, such as CD8[+] PCAETCL or primary cutaneous gamma-delta T-cell lymphomas (**Fig. 7**).[28] The former is a rare CTCL subtype that clinically manifests as rapidly progressing and widely distributed serpiginous patches, plaques, nodules, and tumors, with central necrosis, ulceration, and crustation in elderly patients. The distribution is generalized, but extensive acral and mucosal involvement may be observed.[29] Uncommonly, this condition may manifest with hyperkerathotic or verrucous crusted nodules or plaques, which individually may resemble a generalized form of PR. The epidermotropism of medium-sized cells tends to be massive in CD8[+] PCAETCL with variable necrotic keratinocytes, ulceration, and secondary mixed inflammation. An important clue to reach this diagnosis is the frequent involvement of pilosebaceous and/or eccrine structures. The malignant infiltrate of medium-sized atypical lymphocytes may extend into the deep dermis arranged in a nodular or diffuse pattern.[29] CD8 expression is the only constant finding of this aggressive CTCL variant, but cells are also mostly CD3, CD7, CD45RA, βF-1, and CD45RO and CD30 mostly negative (**Fig. 8**). These cases carry an aggressive clinical course with a 5-year survival of 18% of the cases.[29] The only reports of prolonged survival have been cases of treatment with allogeneic stem cell transplantation.

The clinical presentation of corrugated, hyperkeratotic, or even eroded plaques, besides the high expression of CD30 found in some PR biopsies, occasionally associated with pseudoepitheliomatous hyperplasia, may lead to misdiagnosis with as CD30[+] lymphoproliferative disorder. Type D LyP is a rare subtype of LyP characterized by marked pagetoid epidermotropism of small to medium-sized CD8[+] cells, in contrast with the large cells and lesser epidermotropism typically seen in conventional LyP. All those cases, however, clinically showed typical lesions of LyP.

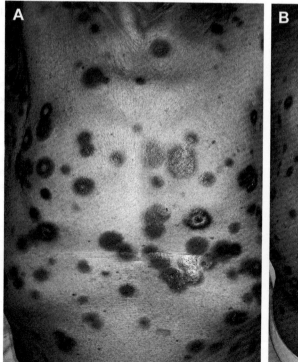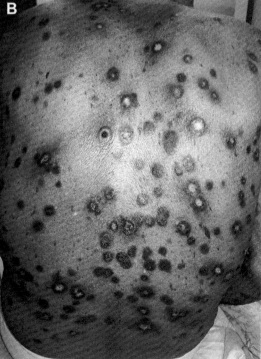

Fig. 7. Two views (*A, B*) of a clinical manifestation of CD8[+] PCAETCL, characterized by multiple erythematous and brownish plaques with central ulceration. Such cases were previously classified as a generalized form of PR (Ketron-Goodman type) but are now considered to represent other types of CTCL.

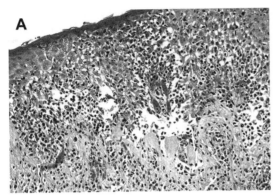
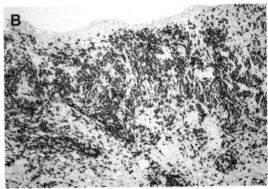

Fig. 8. Histologic features of CD8⁺ PCAETCL. (*A*) Prominent epidermotropism of atypical lymphocytes with clear halo (HE, original magnification ×20). (*B*) Strong CD8⁺ expression is observed in the intraepidermal lymphocytes (HE, original magnification ×10).

Finally, a differential diagnosis with Acral pseudolymphomatous angiokeratoma of children (APACHE) may be considered in certain PR cases presenting in childhood. APACHE is a rare disorder considered a cutaneous pseudolymphoma and is characterized by unilateral erythematous eruption with multiple angiomatous papules on acral areas, mainly in children. Histologically, it shows a dense infiltrate immediately beneath the epidermis and thick-walled vessels. The lymphocytic infiltrate shows a CD4:CD8 ratio of 1:1, few B cells, and reactive features.[19]

△△ Differential Diagnosis
OF PAGETOID RETICULOSIS

A. Inflammatory or infectious skin disease (clinically)
- Eczema
- Psoriasiform dermatitis
- Tuberculosa verrucosa cutis
- Blastomycosis
- Leishmania
- Tinea (dermatophyte infection)
- Verruca vulgaris

B. Skin cancer (non-CTCL)
- Squamous cell carcinoma (clinically and histologically)
- Melanoma (histologically, also when associated to pseudopeitheliomatous hyperplasia)

C. Other types of CTCL and pseudolymphomas
- Unilesional MF
- MF palmaris et plantaris
- CD8⁺ PCAETCL
- Cutaneous CD30⁺ lymphoproliferative disorders (type D LyP)
- APACHE (may be considered when presenting in childhood)

PROGNOSIS

Skin-directed therapies, including topical steroids, topical nitrogen mustard, PUVA, narrow-band UVB (NB-UVB), radiation therapy, and surgery, are reported as treatment options for this condition. In the authors' experience, localized electron-beam therapy is most effective for solitary or limited areas, especially for thick plaques with marked verrucous hyperplasia.[30] Such thick lesions are not amenable to other skin-directed therapies.

PR has an indolent clinical behavior. Recurrence and relapses, however, are frequent either at the original or at a separate site but have little propensity to dissemination or extracutaneous involvement.[30,31]

GRANULOMATOUS SLACK SKIN SYNDROME

OVERVIEW

GSSS is an unusual form of CTCL and also considered a distinct MF variant by the WHO classification.[4,32] As implied by its name, GSSS presents in flexural folds with redundant skin with poor elasticity and a granulomatous infiltrate with elastolysis and multinucleated giant cells. Until now, fewer than 50 cases, including a few small case series, have been published. The rarity of this condition

Key Histologic Features
OF GRANULOMATOUS SLACK SKIN SYNDROM

Main feature: interstitial atypical lymphocytic infiltrate through entire dermis with ill-defined granulomatous changes

Other features

- Variable epidermotropism

- Multinucleated giant cells with 20–30 nuclei/cell

- Variable emperipolesis

- Loss of elastic fibers (elastic Van Gieson stain)

Immunophenotype

- $CD3^+$, $CD4^+$,$CD8^-$; or $CD3^+$, $CD4^-$, $CD8^+$

is exemplified by the largest series comprising only 4 patients.[33–35]

CLINICAL FEATURES

GSSS first presents with the development of ill-defined erythematous infiltrative patches and plaques that typically evolve to bulky, indurated plaques covered by atrophic skin in the flexural areas (axilla and inguinal folds).[33,36] Over time, elasticity is lost, with the appearance of redundant skin evolving into pendulous folds. Skin lesions can also involve other parts of the body; however, loss of elasticity or cutis laxa–like changes in those areas is less prominent. Granulomatous lymphadenitis has been described as an extracutaneous site of involvement, although this finding is exceedingly rare. Pulmonary and splenic noncaseating granulomas have been reported in 2 patients, one of whom died from non-Hodgkin lymphoma.[35] In addition, a second patient developed a primary cutaneous $CD30^+$ lymphoproliferative disorder.[33] These reports raised concerns about the nature of GSSS in relation to other lymphoproliferative conditions. Could GSSS be merely a clinicopathologic event associated with other primary lymphomas? Or is the GSSS association with other lymphoid malignancies a reflection of an increased predisposition to lymphomas in general? These questions are difficult to answer because of the extreme rarity of this condition. The male-to-female ratio seems increased (2.9:1), and the age of onset is wide ranging from childhood to elderly.

DIAGNOSIS: MICROSCOPIC FEATURES

The histologic features of GSSS are characterized by a diffuse infiltrate throughout the entire dermis of small to medium-sized lymphocytes, more commonly with interstitial granulomatous changes and scattered multinucleated giant cells.[37] Multinucleated giant cells displaying between 20 and 30 nuclei per cell is considered a pathognomonic feature.[38,39] The engulfment of lymphocytes (emperiploiesis) and elastic fibers is often observed.

DIAGNOSIS: ANCILLARY STUDIES

Neoplastic T-cell lymphocytes can display a $CD3^+$ $CD4^+$ $CD8^-$, or less commonly $CD3^+$ $CD4^-CD8^+$ phenotype. Verhoeff-van Gieson staining demonstrates loss of elastic fibers within the papillary and reticular dermis. TCR gene rearrangement reviewed in the literature was detected in 8 of 13 of published cases.[33,35]

DIFFERENTIAL DIAGNOSIS

In advanced GSSS, the skin lesions are so characteristic that a diagnosis can be achieved based purely on clinical grounds. Skin biopsy is always needed, however, to confirm a diagnosis. A diagnosis of early disease is more difficult, because it can be clinically and histologically indistinguishable from other variants of CTCL, which also often involves intertriginous areas.

Granulomatous MF, interstitial MF, and cutis laxa–like MF are MF variants that may resemble early phases of GSSS.[40] The authors think that all these MF variants, including GSSS, should be considered in the same spectrum with variable clinicopathologic presentation based on the stage of evolution and in all cases representing an immune granulomatous response against the neoplastic T cells. Granulomatous MF is manifested as erythematous, violaceous to hyperpigmented patches/plaques, granuloma annulare–like lesions, or hyperkeratotic plaques that do not evolve into cutis laxa–like features. Histologic features are characterized by dermal infiltrates that may range from patchy to dense and may extend through the entire dermis, with focal epidermotropism and a lichenoid component. Histiocytes may arrange in sarcoidal aggregates or a more diffuse interstitial pattern intermingled with the neoplastic T-cell infiltrate (**Fig. 9**A–C). Multinucleated giant cells, as well as elastophagocytosis, may be rarely observed. Thus, granulomatous MF may histopathologically overlap with GSSS, and clinical correlation is needed for classification. The atypical lymphocytic infiltrate is commonly

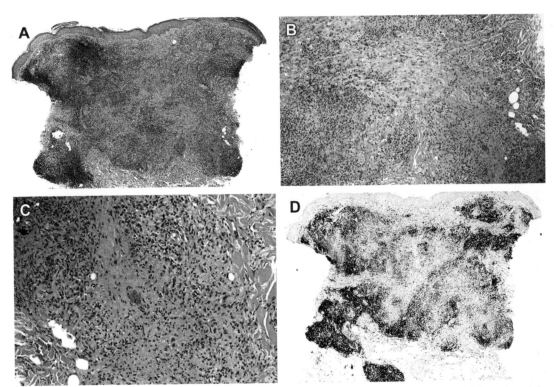

Fig. 9. Histologic features of granulomatous MF. (*A*) Low power. Moderately dense, interstitial, and nodular dermal infiltrate (HE, original magnification ×2). (*B, C*) High-power view showing prominent histiocytes and lymphocytes (HE, original magnification ×10), (HE, original magnification ×20). (*D*) The atypical lymphocytic infiltrate in this case is predominantly CD8$^+$ (original magnification ×2).

CD8$^+$ and rarely CD4$^+$ (see **Fig. 9**D). In the authors' experience, patients with CD8$^+$ granulomatous CTCL tend to present with deep infiltrated plaques and nodules with constitutional symptoms and frequent involvement of lung and pleura. This presentation may overlap or closely resemble granulomatous reactions observed in associated with primary (eg, Burton syndrome or ataxia-telangiectasia) or secondary (iatrogenic) immunodeficiency (**Fig. 10**).

Interstitial MF is a rare variant characterized by a dermal infiltrate composed of predominantly lymphocytes with few histiocytes between collagen bundles, without destruction of elastic fibers, at least during the early phase or at the time of diagnosis (**Fig. 11**).[41] It is clinically manifested as erythematous ill-defined patches or plaques, with or without pruritus, and occasionally resembling granuloma annulare or inflammatory morphea (**Fig. 12**). The authors suggest that some cases of interstitial MF, especially a common presentation involving intertriginous areas, might represent an early stage of GSSS. The cutis laxa–like phase may be avoided once remission is achieved with early intervention. An extremely rare case of cutis

laxa–like MF has been reported, showing generalized wrinkled skin on the trunk and extremities without involvement of skin folds. Skin biopsy showed an atrophic epidermis with similar histologic changes seen in GSSS.[40]

In addition, granulomatous features can be found in other types of CTCL, such as FMF. As discussed previously, a granulomatous reaction is often observed in association with lymphomatous disruption of the follicular epithelium with exposure of keratin material to the adjacent dermis. Other CTCL subtypes have been reported to occasionally display granulomatous changes, including Sézary syndrome, primary cutaneous anaplastic large cell lymphoma, and subcutaneous panniculitis–like T-cell lymphoma.[33,42]

Another differential diagnosis that should be included is acquired cutis laxa, which is an acquired connective tissue disorder characterized by loose, hanging, and wrinkled skin folds with loss of elasticity. It commonly affects face, shoulders, and thighs, and it is clinically more subtle than the skin folds that are seen in GSSS. Histologically, the atypical lymphocytic infiltrate is missing.

△△ Differential Diagnosis
OF GRANULOMATOUS SLACK SKIN SYNDROME

- Acquired cutis laxa syndrome
- Granulomatous MF
- Interstitial MF
- Cutis laxa–like MF
- Other types of CTCL that may present granulomatous histologic features: FMF, Sézary syndrome, cutaneous anaplastic large cell lymphoma, and subcutaneous panniculitis–like T-cell lymphoma

PROGNOSIS

There is no specific therapeutic regimen for GSSS, and the treatment options used in the literature are those considered for CTCL in general. Complete response has never been reported, although partial response has been achieved with PUVA, radiation therapy, chemotherapy, systemic steroids, azathioprine, interferon (α and γ), surgery, and some combination therapies.[43]

GSSS has a slowly progressive course with rare cases developing nodal involvement, but even these more extensive cases seem to follow an indolent course with prolonged survival.[44]

HYPOPIGMENTED MYCOSIS FUNGOIDES

Key Histologic Features
OF HYPOPIGMENTED MF

Main feature: epidermotropic lymphocytic infiltrate with a predilection for the basal cell layer

Other features

- Atypia confined to intraepidermal compartment
- Mild reactive lymphoid infiltrate in dermis
- Melanin-laden macrophages in upper dermis

Immunophenotype

- CD3$^+$, CD4$^-$, CD8$^+$ or occasionally CD3$^+$, CD4$^+$, CD8$^-$
- Loss of CD7

OVERVIEW

HMF is one of several clinicopathologic variants of MF not yet recognized by the WHO classification. First described by Ryan and colleagues[45] in 1973, with several case series published since then, this variant tends to affect children and young patients and has been reported more often in patients with

Fig. 10. Clinical presentation of granulomatous MF associated with immunodeficiency. (*A, B*) Multiple erythematous and scaly nonconfluent papules and nodules on the back.

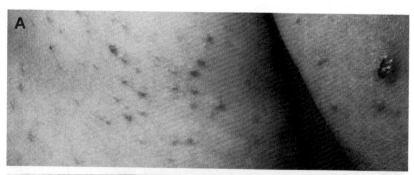

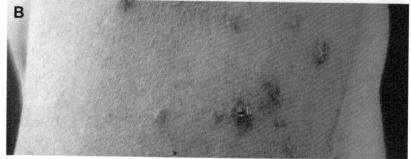

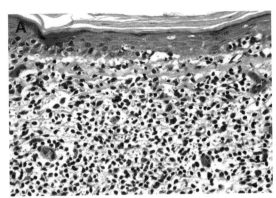
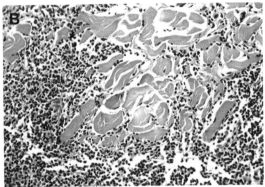

Fig. 11. Histologic findings in interstitial MF. (A) Atrophic epidermis with vacuolization of the basal layer, with scattered intraepidermal lymphocytes and lichenoid infiltrate of atypical lymphocytes (HE, original magnification ×40). (B) Atypical lymphocytic infiltrate within the dermal collagen bundles (HE, original magnification ×20).

dark complexion.[46,47] White patients rarely are reported.[46] Based on the markedly indolent course frequently noted and the poor histologic criteria in some of the published cases, the authors think that HMF may be overdiagnosed. Such cases of dubious histology, positive T-cell clonality, and indolent course may represent hypopigmented variants of CLD rather than CTCL.[16]

CLINICAL FEATURES

Patients with HMF manifest asymmetric hypopigmented patches or plaques in a wide distribution of sites (Figs. 13 and 14). Although several investigators consider HMF a form of CTCL in which hypopigmentation occurs in the absence of classic lesions of MF, others suggest that HMF can coexist with erythematous patches, plaques, or tumors more typical of conventional MF.[46] This mixed clinical pattern (hypopigmented and erythematous) is predominantly reported in white patients, in which HMF seems rare. Subtle erythematous lesions, however, may be difficult to identify in dark-skinned individuals.[46]

DIAGNOSIS: MICROSCOPIC FEATURES

Microscopically, one of the most salient features is the presence of atypical cells almost exclusively involving the intraepidermal compartment, with a predilection for infiltration along the basal cell layer. Skin biopsies typically show an epidermotropic lymphocytic infiltrate of CD8+ slightly pleomorphic, medium-sized lymphocytes along the basal cell layer in a pattern resembling a string of pearls (Fig. 15A). Pautrier microabscesses or marked pagetoid spread are rarely observed. The dermis often shows a reactive lymphoid infiltrate with melanin-laden macrophages, and adnexal structures are for the most part free of involvement.

DIAGNOSIS: ANCILLARY STUDIES

Immunohistochemical analysis shows a predominantly CD8+ infiltrate (see Fig. 15B), however, a CD4+ phenotype can be observed. Atypical lymphocytes occasionally show loss of CD7.[46,47] TCR gene rearrangement is frequently detected

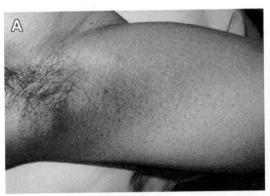
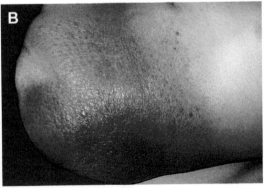

Fig. 12. Interstitial MF. (A) Erythematous, brownish, slightly scaly patch in axillary area. (B) Erythematous, violaceous patch on the left flank.

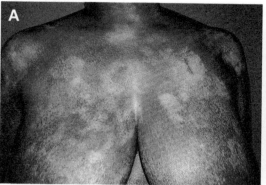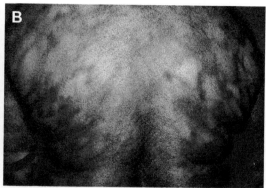

Fig. 13. (*A, B*) HMF presenting with extensive confluent, asymmetric, dyschromic patches.

even in cases of limited disease and very innocuous course.[16,48]

DIFFERENTIAL DIAGNOSIS

The differential diagnoses in HMF includes inflammatory dermatoses, such as vitiligo, pityriasis alba, pityriasis lichenoides chronica, progressive macular hypomelanosis, sarcoidosis, and postinflammatory hypopigmentation.[46,47] In addition, infectious skin diseases, such as leprosy, tinea versicolor, syphilis, and onchocerciasis, should be considered in certain situations.[47] The authors, however, consider that the most difficult differential diagnosis of HMF is with the hypopigmented variant of CLD. The clinical evolution may be helpful in the diagnosis, with a prolonged,

nonaggressive course and response to conventional treatments, preferably NB-UVB, and eventual resolution of the lesions with normal pigmentation after regression of the infiltrate.[46]

PROGNOSIS

HMF has been reported to follow an indolent course, especially in children.[49,50] This observation suggests the possibility that some cases may have been improperly classified as lymphomas and that a CLD could have been considered. Other HMF cases, especially the ones with mixed lesions, show a similar course of patch-stage conventional MF with survival based on stage and tumor burden.[46,47] The lesions tend to persist for a long time but respond well to phototherapy or topical chemotherapy, with resolution of the lesions and eventual repigmentation. Persistent dyschromia, however, may occur in some cases.

OTHER RARE VARIANTS OF MF

Syringotropic MF is characterized by an atypical lymphocytic infiltrate that is located mainly in the deep dermis, around and within hyperplastic eccrine sweat gland coils. This variant often overlaps with FMF and may present with alopecia, a punctuate erythematous process, or ill-defined patches associated with hypohidrosis or anhidrosis. Erythematous scaly patches with or without a papular component involving palms and soles are also highly suspicious for this variant of MF (**Fig. 16**). Histologically, dense perieccrine infiltrates of small to medium-sized cerebriform cells invading the secretory and to a lesser extent the ductal portions of eccrine glands are the defining pathology. Epithelial hyperplasia of the eccrine coil may be noted. Focal perieccrine involvement also is seen in classical MF, but in such cases

---

△△ **Differential Diagnosis**
OF HYPOPIGMENTED MF

A. Inflammatory dermatoses
- Vitiligo
- Pityriasis alba
- Pityriasis lichenoides chronica
- Progressive macular hypomelanosis
- Sarcoidosis
- Postinflammatory hyperpigmentation

B. Infectious skin diseases
- Leprosy
- Tinea versicolor
- Syphilis
- Onchocerciasis

C. CLD

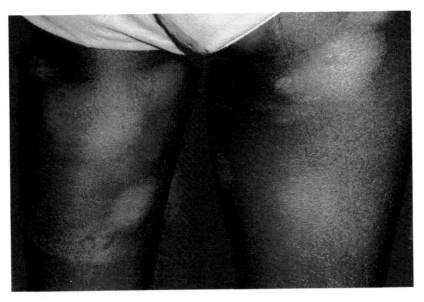

Fig. 14. HMF in a child. Hypopigmented and well-demarcated patches, some with annular pattern localized on bilateral posterior thighs.

the infiltrate is less prominent and without infiltration of the glandular epithelium. Epidermotropism is uncommon, and Pautrier microabscesses are usually absent. Hair follicles may be concurrently involved or even destroyed by the neoplastic infiltrate. Therefore, adnexotropic MF could be a more accurate term for such cases. The differential diagnosis may include syringolymphoid hyperplasia with alopecia, which may represent a CLD and usually manifests with a single or few patches of alopecia with anhidrosis.

Pigmented purpuric-like MF is manifested with a purpuric hue with golden brown discoloration simulating true pigmented purpuric dermatoses (PPD). Concomitant lesions of classical MF may be present, helping to reach a diagnosis. Histologically, extravasated erythrocytes within the infiltrate of atypical lymphocytes along the superficial dermis with a lichenoid pattern and some epidermotropism are characteristic. Hemosiderin deposition is also frequently noted. The main differential diagnosis is with lichen aureus and other pigmented purpuric dermatosis, which are often associated with clonal TCR gene rearrangement. Lichen aureus should have limited clinical involvement, typically on the lower

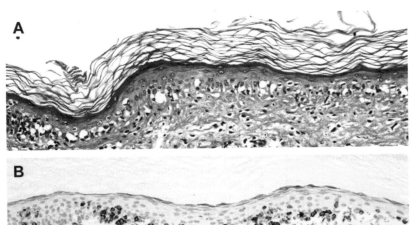

Fig. 15. Histologic features of HMF. (*A*) Atypical lymphocytes with a string of pearls–like arrangement along the basal cell layer (HE, original magnification ×20). (*B*) The atypical lymphocytes are CD8[+] (original magnification ×20).

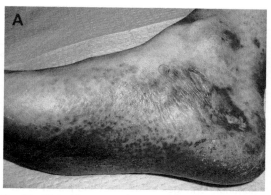
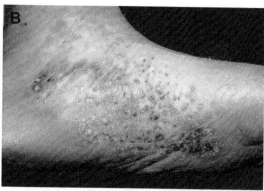

Fig. 16. Clinical features of syringotropic MF. (*A, B*) A papular erythematous eruption localized in the inner area of bilateral soles.

extremities, and histologically lacking significant lymphoid atypia. The authors think that cases of PPD with T-cell clonality and chronic recalcitrant course should be considered a CLD subtype, assuming that the histopathology is not consistent with MF.[51,52] Nonetheless, close follow-up of these patients is warranted.

Poikilodermatous MF is a variant that manifests in a substantial number of patients with an otherwise typical clinical picture of MF who may develop poikilodermic-type lesions, characterized by dyschromia with hypo- and hyperpigmentation, dryness, atrophy, and telangiectasia (poikiloderma atrophicans vasculare) (**Fig. 17**). These lesions often develop at the sites of preexisting patches and can be associated with typical patches and plaques of MF elsewhere. Additional histopathologic changes typical of poikiloderma include atrophy of the epidermis with flattening or loss of rete ridges, subtle to moderate vacuolar alteration of the basal layer, and dilatation of superficial blood vessels containing erythrocytes.[53]

Papular MF is a controversial entity and may be considered a manifestation of early MF with erythematous, nonpruritic, and chronic papules distributed on the trunk and extremities, without classical erythematous patches typically seen in classical MF. Gender predominance was not seen in 10 cases reported, and the age of onset ranged from 31 to 63 years. An epidermotropic infiltrate of predominantly CD4$^+$ T cells is observed histologically. Differential diagnosis includes nonspecific folliculitis, pityriasis lichenoides, lichen nitidus, and most importantly type B LyP, which may be clinically and pathologically indistinguishable. This rare type of LyP differs from papular MF by its typical waxing and waning course and the tendency to present in clusters. Based on a few case reports, papular MF seems to have a good prognosis and usually responds to skin-directed treatments used in early MF.[54]

Bullous/vesicular MF is manifested mostly in elderly people as flaccid or tense, often multiple or even generalized blisters appearing either on

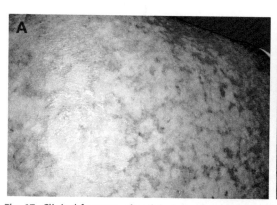
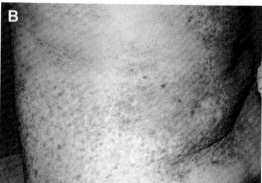

Fig. 17. Clinical features of poikilodermatous MF. (*A*) Hypo- and hyperpigmentation associated with telangiectasias on the back of a 69-year-old woman. (*B*) Hypo- and hyperpigmented confluent plaques localized on the trunk of 43-year-old woman.

normal skin, on an erythematous base, or within typical plaques and tumors of MF. Histologically, all common features of MF (epidermotropism, atypical lymphocytes, and so forth) are seen, and blisters may occur in various locations (subcorneal, intraepidermal, and subepidermal). The differential diagnosis with impetiginized and severe spongiotic eczematous conditions and with immunobullous diseases may be difficult and may require close follow-up with multiple biopsies as well as TCR gene rearrangement analysis and immunofluorescence studies.[55]

Vegetating/papillomatous MF (also referred to as acanthosis nigricans–like) is an extremely rare MF variant characterized by hyperkeratotic and sometimes hyperpigmented patches or plaques that arise in flexural areas (axillae and groin), neck, and breast (nipple and areolae). The lesions may clinically resemble acanthosis nigricans depending on their configuration, size, and color. Histologically, there is papillomatosis, marked acanthosis, and a bandlike or diffuse infiltrate of atypical lymphocytes.[56]

Ichthyosiform MF is a rare subtype that presents clinically as widespread ichthyosiform lesions often accompanied by comedo-like lesions and/or follicular keratotic papules. Although the ichthyosiform changes are usually the only manifestations of this MF variant, the combination of classical MF and acquired ichthyosis (as a paraneoplastic phenomenon) has been documented. Histologically, the ichthyosiform areas demonstrate compact orthokeratosis, hypogranulosis, and a bandlike epidermotropic infiltrate composed of small cerebriform lymphocytes (**Fig. 18**).[57]

Lichenoid MF is a rare variant that presents with histopathologic features of a lichenoid tissue reaction (LTR) in the skin biopsy. LTR is characterized by the presence of epidermal basal cell damage that is associated with a bandlike infiltrate of mononuclear cells in the upper dermis and squamatization of the basal cell layer. A case series of 12 patients showed a wide range of clinical manifestations, with pruritus and/or a burning sensation the most consistent finding. The atypical lymphocytic infiltrate was predominantly CD4+. Half of the patients showed disease progression; thus, lichenoid changes in MF were suggested to carry a poor prognosis. Differential diagnosis should include other lichenoid conditions, such as extensive lichen planus.[58]

Invisible MF is a term that has been used to define several cases of normal-looking skin and persistent pruritus that showed histologic features of MF. Pruritus is not usually present in MF in the absence of cutaneous lesions but has occasionally been reported to precede the disease for as long as 10 years.[59] The authors have observed recurrent MF presenting with pruritus and without obvious skin lesions but noted, however, that subtle ill-defined erythema became more obvious when photographs with flash were taken.

In conclusion, the authors have reviewed several clinicopathologic variants of MF. Some of them are formally recognized in the 2008 WHO classification, whereas others have been reported in the literature but not yet accepted as distinct entities or variants. The classification of cutaneous lymphomas is often said to be a "work in progress" endeavor that evolves and

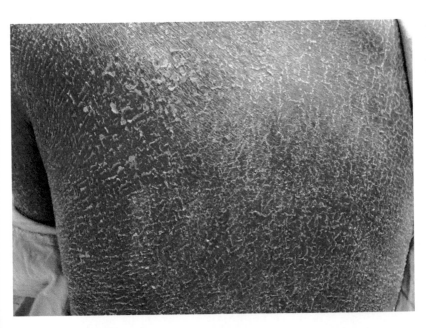

Fig. 18. Clinical features of ichthyosiform MF. Diffuse scaly and confluent plaques with erythematous background.

changes as more is learned about the spectrum of cutaneous lymphoproliferative disorders. The authors foresee continued expansion, refinement, and improvement of classification schemes to help comprehend the extent and complexity of these challenging conditions.

REFERENCES

1. Kazakov DV, Burg G, Kempf W. Clinicopathological spectrum of mycosis fungoides. J Eur Acad Dermatol Venereol 2004;18(4):397–415.

2. Lessin SR. Alibert lymphoma: renaming mycosis fungoides. Arch Dermatol 2009;145(2):209–10.

3. Nashan D, Faulhaber D, Stander S, et al. Mycosis fungoides: a dermatological masquerader. Br J Dermatol 2007;156(1):1–10.

4. Willemze R, Jaffe ES, Burg G, et al. WHO-EORTC classification for cutaneous lymphomas. Blood 2005;105(10):3768–85.

5. Gerami P, Rosen S, Kuzel T, et al. Folliculotropic mycosis fungoides: an aggressive variant of cutaneous T-cell lymphoma. Arch Dermatol 2008; 144(6):738–46.

6. van Doorn R, Scheffer E, Willemze R. Follicular mycosis fungoides, a distinct disease entity with or without associated follicular mucinosis: a clinicopathologic and follow-up study of 51 patients. Arch Dermatol 2002;138(2):191–8.

7. Shin J, Monti S, Aires DJ, et al. Lesional gene expression profiling in cutaneous T-cell lymphoma reveals natural clusters associated with disease outcome. Blood 2007;110(8):3015–27.

8. Gerami P, Guitart J. The spectrum of histopathologic and immunohistochemical findings in folliculotropic mycosis fungoides. Am J Surg Pathol 2007; 31(9):1430–8.

9. Lehman JS, Cook-Norris RH, Weed BR, et al. Folliculotropic mycosis fungoides: single-center study and systematic review. Arch Dermatol 2010; 146(6):607–13.

10. Ruiz-Genao D, Ballestero M, Fraga J, et al. Follicular mycosis fungoides, comedo-like and cystic. Actas Dermosifiliogr 2005;96(2):102–5 [in Spanish].

11. Alikhan A, Griffin J, Nguyen N, et al. Pediatric follicular mucinosis: presentation, histopathology, molecular genetics, treatment, and outcomes over an 11-year period at the Mayo Clinic. Pediatr Dermatol 2013;30(2):192–8.

12. Cerroni L, Fink-Puches R, Back B, et al. Follicular mucinosis: a critical reappraisal of clinicopathologic features and association with mycosis fungoides and Sezary syndrome. Arch Dermatol 2002;138(2):182–9.

13. Gibson LE, Muller SA, Peters MS. Follicular mucinosis of childhood and adolescence. Pediatr Dermatol 1988;5(4):231–5.

14. Jackow CM, Papadopoulos E, Nelson B, et al. Follicular mucinosis associated with scarring alopecia, oligoclonal T-cell receptor V beta expansion, and Staphylococcus aureus: when does follicular mucinosis become mycosis fungoides? J Am Acad Dermatol 1997;37(5 Pt 2):828–31.

15. Flaig MJ, Cerroni L, Schuhmann K, et al. Follicular mycosis fungoides. A histopathologic analysis of nine cases. J Cutan Pathol 2001;28(10):525–30.

16. Guitart J, Magro C. Cutaneous T-cell lymphoid dyscrasia: a unifying term for idiopathic chronic dermatoses with persistent T-cell clones. Arch Dermatol 2007;143(7):921–32.

17. Muniesa C, Estrach T, Pujol RM, et al. Folliculotropic mycosis fungoides: clinicopathological features and outcome in a series of 20 cases. J Am Acad Dermatol 2010;62(3):418–26.

18. Agar NS, Wedgeworth E, Crichton S, et al. Survival outcomes and prognostic factors in mycosis fungoides/Sezary syndrome: validation of the revised International Society for Cutaneous Lymphomas/European Organisation for Research and Treatment of Cancer staging proposal. J Clin Oncol 2010;28(31):4730–9.

19. Matsuzaki Y, Kimura K, Nakano H, et al. Localized pagetoid reticulosis (Woringer-Kolopp disease) in early childhood. J Am Acad Dermatol 2009;61(1): 120–3.

20. Mielke V, Wolff HH, Winzer M, et al. Localized and disseminated pagetoid reticulosis. Diagnostic immunophenotypical findings. Arch Dermatol 1989; 125(3):402–6.

21. Steffen C. Ketron-Goodman disease, Woringer-Kolopp disease, and pagetoid reticulosis. Am J Dermatopathol 2005;27(1):68–85.

22. Oliver GF, Winkelmann RK. Unilesional mycosis fungoides: a distinct entity. J Am Acad Dermatol 1989;20(1):63–70.

23. Haghighi B, Smoller BR, LeBoit PE, et al. Pagetoid reticulosis (Woringer-Kolopp disease): an immunophenotypic, molecular, and clinicopathologic study. Mod Pathol 2000;13(5):502–10.

24. El Shabrawi-Caelen L, Cerroni L, Kerl H. The clinicopathologic spectrum of cytotoxic lymphomas of the skin. Semin Cutan Med Surg 2000;19(2): 118–23.

25. Mourtzinos N, Puri PK, Wang G, et al. CD4/CD8 double negative pagetoid reticulosis: a case report and literature review. J Cutan Pathol 2010;37(4): 491–6.

26. Jacyk WK, Grayson W, Dinkel JE, et al. Pagetoid reticulosis with CD30 positivity and cytotoxic/suppressor cells. J Cutan Pathol 2007;34(8):644–7.

27. Kim ST, Jeon YS, Sim HJ, et al. Clinicopathologic features and T-cell receptor gene rearrangement findings of mycosis fungoides palmaris et plantaris. J Am Acad Dermatol 2006;54(3):466–71.

28. Berti E, Tomasini D, Vermeer MH, et al. Primary cutaneous CD8-positive epidermotropic cytotoxic T cell lymphomas. A distinct clinicopathological entity with an aggressive clinical behavior. Am J Pathol 1999;155(2):483–92.

29. Nofal A, Abdel-Mawla MY, Assaf M, et al. Primary cutaneous aggressive epidermotropic CD8+ T-cell lymphoma: proposed diagnostic criteria and therapeutic evaluation. J Am Acad Dermatol 2012;67(4):748–59.

30. Lee J, Viakhireva N, Cesca C, et al. Clinicopathologic features and treatment outcomes in Woringer-Kolopp disease. J Am Acad Dermatol 2008;59(4):706–12.

31. Burns MK, Chan LS, Cooper KD. Woringer-Kolopp disease (localized pagetoid reticulosis) or unilesional mycosis fungoides? An analysis of eight cases with benign disease. Arch Dermatol 1995; 131(3):325–9.

32. Burg G, Kempf W, Kazakov DV, et al. Cutaneous lymphomas. Boca Raton (FL): Taylor & Francis; 2005.

33. Kempf W, Ostheeren-Michaelis S, Paulli M, et al. Granulomatous mycosis fungoides and granulomatous slack skin: a multicenter study of the Cutaneous Lymphoma Histopathology Task Force Group of the European Organization For Research and Treatment of Cancer (EORTC). Arch Dermatol 2008;144(12):1609–17.

34. van Haselen CW, Toonstra J, van der Putte SJ, et al. Granulomatous slack skin. Report of three patients with an updated review of the literature. Dermatology 1998;196(4):382–91.

35. Gadzia J, Kestenbaum T. Granulomatous slack skin without evidence of a clonal T-cell proliferation. J Am Acad Dermatol 2004;50(2 Suppl):S4–8.

36. LeBoit PE. Granulomatous slack skin. Dermatol Clin 1994;12(2):375–89.

37. Rongioletti F, Cerroni L, Massone C, et al. Different histologic patterns of cutaneous granulomas in systemic lymphoma. J Am Acad Dermatol 2004;51(4):600–5.

38. Clarijs M, Poot F, Laka A, et al. Granulomatous slack skin: treatment with extensive surgery and review of the literature. Dermatology 2003;206(4):393–7.

39. LeBoit PE, Zackheim HS, White CR Jr. Granulomatous variants of cutaneous T-cell lymphoma. The histopathology of granulomatous mycosis fungoides and granulomatous slack skin. Am J Surg Pathol 1988;12(2):83–95.

40. Lopez Aventin D, Gallardo F, Gil I, et al. Cutis laxa-like mycosis fungoides. J Dermatol 2012;39(6):548–51.

41. Su LD, Kim YH, LeBoit PE, et al. Interstitial mycosis fungoides, a variant of mycosis fungoides resembling granuloma annulare and inflammatory morphea. J Cutan Pathol 2002;29(3):135–41.

42. Scarabello A, Leinweber B, Ardigo M, et al. Cutaneous lymphomas with prominent granulomatous reaction: a potential pitfall in the histopathologic diagnosis of cutaneous T- and B-cell lymphomas. Am J Surg Pathol 2002;26(10):1259–68.

43. Teixeira M, Alves R, Lima M, et al. Granulomatous slack skin. Eur J Dermatol 2007;17(5):435–8.

44. Shah A, Safaya A. Granulomatous slack skin disease: a review, in comparison with mycosis fungoides. J Eur Acad Dermatol Venereol 2012; 26(12):1472–8.

45. Ryan EA, Sanderson KV, Bartak P, et al. Can mycosis fungoides begin in the epidermis? A hypothesis. Br J Dermatol 1973;88(5):419–29.

46. Ardigo M, Borroni G, Muscardin L, et al. Hypopigmented mycosis fungoides in Caucasian patients: a clinicopathologic study of 7 cases. J Am Acad Dermatol 2003;49(2):264–70.

47. El-Shabrawi-Caelen L, Cerroni L, Medeiros LJ, et al. Hypopigmented mycosis fungoides: frequent expression of a CD8+ T-cell phenotype. Am J Surg Pathol 2002;26(4):450–7.

48. Volkenandt M, Soyer HP, Cerroni L, et al. Molecular detection of clone-specific DNA in hypopigmented lesions of a patient with early evolving mycosis fungoides. Br J Dermatol 1993;128(4):423–8.

49. Dummer R, Kamarashev J, Kempf W, et al. Junctional CD8+ cutaneous lymphomas with nonaggressive clinical behavior: a CD8+ variant of mycosis fungoides? Arch Dermatol 2002;138(2):199–203.

50. Whittam LR, Calonje E, Orchard G, et al. CD8-positive juvenile onset mycosis fungoides: an immunohistochemical and genotypic analysis of six cases. Br J Dermatol 2000;143(6):1199–204.

51. Barnhill RL, Braverman IM. Progression of pigmented purpura-like eruptions to mycosis fungoides: report of three cases. J Am Acad Dermatol 1988;19(1 Pt 1):25–31.

52. Viseux V, Schoenlaub P, Cnudde F, et al. Pigmented purpuric dermatitis preceding the diagnosis of mycosis fungoides by 24 years. Dermatology 2003;207(3):331–2.

53. Abbott RA, Sahni D, Robson A, et al. Poikilodermatous mycosis fungoides: a study of its clinicopathological, immunophenotypic, and prognostic features. J Am Acad Dermatol 2011; 65(2):313–9.

54. Kodama K, Fink-Puches R, Massone C, et al. Papular mycosis fungoides: a new clinical variant of early mycosis fungoides. J Am Acad Dermatol 2005;52(4):694–8.

55. Bowman PH, Hogan DJ, Sanusi ID. Mycosis fungoides bullosa: report of a case and review of the literature. J Am Acad Dermatol 2001;45(6):934–9.

56. Willemze R, Scheffer E, Van Vloten WA. Mycosis fungoides simulating acanthosis nigricans. Am J Dermatopathol 1985;7(4):367–71.

57. Marzano AV, Borghi A, Facchetti M, et al. Ichthyosiform mycosis fungoides. Dermatology 2002;204(2): 124–9.

58. Guitart J, Peduto M, Caro WA, et al. Lichenoid changes in mycosis fungoides. J Am Acad Dermatol 1997;36(3 Pt 1):417–22.

59. Pujol RM, Gallardo F, Llistosella E, et al. Invisible mycosis fungoides: a diagnostic challenge. J Am Acad Dermatol 2000;42(2 Pt 2):324–8.

Sézary Syndrome

Agnieszka W. Kubica, MD[a], Mark R. Pittelkow, MD[b],*

KEYWORDS

- Cutaneous T-cell lymphoma • Diagnosis • Erythroderma • Prognosis • Sézary syndrome

KEY POINTS

- Sézary syndrome (SS) is an aggressive variant of cutaneous T-cell lymphoma (CTCL) characterized by erythroderma and a leukemic burden of circulating malignant T cells. Patients present with erythroderma and pruritus and frequently exhibit palmoplantar keratoderma, lymphadenopathy, and nail changes.
- Diagnosis of SS is based on the TNMB staging outlined by the European Organization for Research and Treatment of Cancer/International Society for Cutaneous Lymphomas (EORTC/ISCL) and is characterized by greater than 80% of total body erythema with identification of a significant T-cell lymphocytic leukemic burden, as confirmed by T-cell gene rearrangements, elevated Sézary cell counts, flow cytometry, or an abnormal or clonal mature T-cell immunophenotype.
- Overall survival in patients with SS ranges from 2.5 to 5 years. Novel molecular data have established potential markers for diagnosis, monitoring of clinical progression, and prognosis for patients with SS.

ABSTRACT

Sézary syndrome (SS), a type of cutaneous T-cell lymphoma with a poor prognosis, is characterized by erythroderma and leukemic involvement. Because of the rarity of SS and difficulty in diagnosis, data on this aggressive malignancy are scarce. In this review, the diagnosis and pathology of SS are summarized and an update is provided, highlighting microscopic features and novel molecular findings. The diagnostic challenge of SS is described, with an emphasis on the differential diagnosis of erythroderma and key points in distinguishing SS from other cutaneous T-cell malignancies. Finally, the prognosis is discussed, focusing on large, recent studies of SS patients.

OVERVIEW

SS is a rare, aggressive leukemic variant of primary CTCL. SS has classically been characterized by a population of mature circulating leukemic T cells in the setting of erythroderma.[1–3] Although SS is a rare malignancy, the incidence of CTCL continues to increase, thus heightening the importance of early, appropriate diagnosis and treatment.[4] The incidence of CTCL has recently been estimated to be between 6.4 and 7.7 cases per 1 million persons,[4,5] with incidence rising over the past 3 decades.[4] Specifically, the incidence of SS was 0.1 to 0.3 cases per 1 million persons during the past three decades.[4,5] Men are affected approximately twice as frequently as women.[4–8] Among all forms of CTCL in general, the black population has a greater incidence, whereas in SS, the incidence is higher in the white population.[4,5] SS incidence increases with age,[1] with the median age at the time of diagnosis in the seventh decade of life.[1,4,6,9–11]

Because the differential diagnosis of erythroderma is large and protean, SS presents a diagnostic challenge that has recently been aided by national and international collaborative initiatives to create a more uniform consensus for diagnosis,

Disclosure Statement: No financial or industry disclosures.
a Department of Dermatology, Mayo Clinic, 200 First Street SW, Rochester, MN 55905, USA; b Department of Dermatology, Mayo Clinic, 13400 East Shea Boulevard, Scottsdale, AZ 85259, USA
* Corresponding author.
E-mail address: pittelkow.mark@mayo.edu

Surgical Pathology 7 (2014) 191–202
http://dx.doi.org/10.1016/j.path.2014.02.005

surgpath.theclinics.com

staging, and treatment, with particular emphasis on identifying new molecular markers and establishing consensus on their diagnostic utility and potential prognostic value. In this review, the clinical features and diagnosis of SS are outlined, with a focus on novel molecular criteria and recent research advances. Subsequently, differential diagnosis and prognosis of SS are discussed, highlighting the challenges of diagnosing and treating this unique and aggressive hematologic and dermatologic malignancy.

CLINICAL FEATURES

SS often presents with protean clinical features, but the key signs and symptoms point to this aggressive mature T-cell malignant lymphoproliferative disorder as the cause. Among the varied signs and symptoms, the physical finding necessary for diagnosis is erythroderma. Erythroderma is defined as erythema that covers 80% or more of the body surface area.

In addition to erythroderma, the other key clinical feature is pruritus, which is almost uniformly present and often severe and refractory to therapy in SS patients.[6,7,12] This symptom is often prominent and incapacitating for SS patients and disrupts daily activities and sleep, but it is seen only rarely in selected types of erythroderma. Pruritus is often widespread, however, and common in various other dermatologic and oncologic conditions. Thus, it is often less helpful diagnostically.

In many patients, lymphadenopathy is evident on careful physical examination, revealing the systemic nature of this malignancy.[6,9,13] A unique and helpful diagnostic clue is the cutaneous finding of palmoplantar keratoderma in SS.[12,14] Nail manifestations include subungual hyperkeratosis, onychomadesis, yellow discoloration, and nail thickening. Other common clinical features are ectropion and alopecia.[6,8,12] In some cases, there may be more extensive lymphoid infiltration of malignant cells accompanied by edema into dermal tissues[15,16] in the form of patches and indurated plaques as well as tumors and the development of a leonine facies.[6,12,17] Representative examples of these physical findings are shown in **Figs. 1–6**. **Box 1** details the common presenting signs and symptoms of SS, and **Box 2** summarizes its key features.

Because of the wide range of presenting symptoms and often insidious development of erythroderma, there is frequently a delay of diagnosis, with clinical series reporting a median duration from onset of initial skin findings or other symptoms to eventual diagnosis of SS of 20.5 months.[12] Recognizing the broad differential diagnosis for erythroderma and other challenges for diagnosis and eventual referral to dermatologists experienced in the diagnosis and treatment of SS, the authors' large institutional experience identified a median delay of 1.7 years from onset of erythroderma to diagnosis, with a range of 0.2 to 7.0 years.[6]

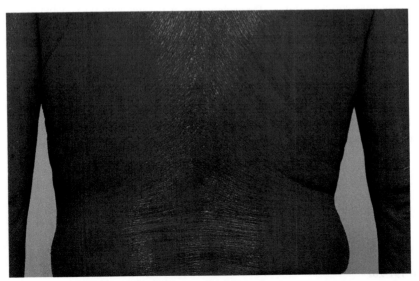

Fig. 1. Erythroderma on the back of a patient with SS.

Fig. 2. Erythroderma with overlying scale and fissuring on the hands and arms of a patient with SS.

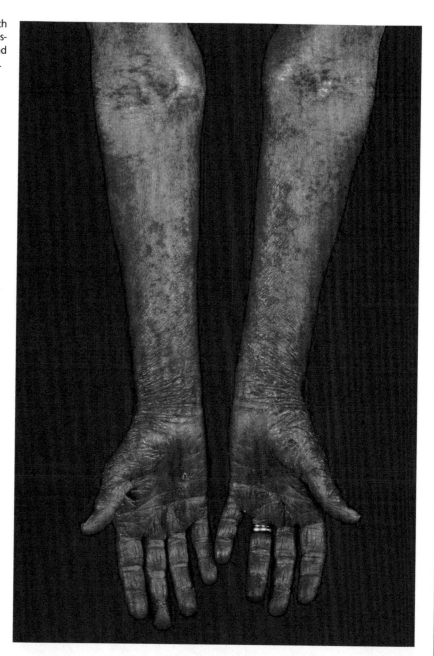

DIAGNOSIS: MICROSCOPIC FEATURES

Whereas skin biopsy specimens of SS patients frequently show a constellation of characteristics that lead to the correct diagnosis, they are not typically pathognomonic and are frequently nonspecific. Overall for CTCL, it has been estimated that only 60% of skin biopsies are diagnostic.[18] Skin biopsies from patients with mycosis fungoides (MF) are more frequently diagnostic than those of SS patients, because absent or minimal epidermotropism is more often noted in SS.[15] As a result of this relative deficiency in diagnostic specificity, skin biopsy interpretation can support or confirm a diagnosis of SS, but histopathologic criteria are not solely diagnostic.

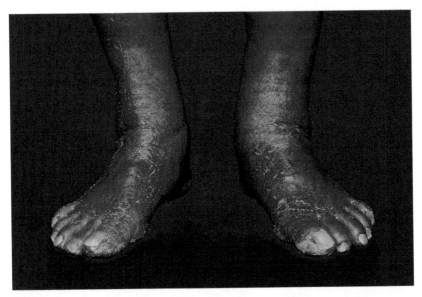

Fig. 3. Erythroderma, hyperkeratosis, and nail dystrophy on the feet of a patient with SS.

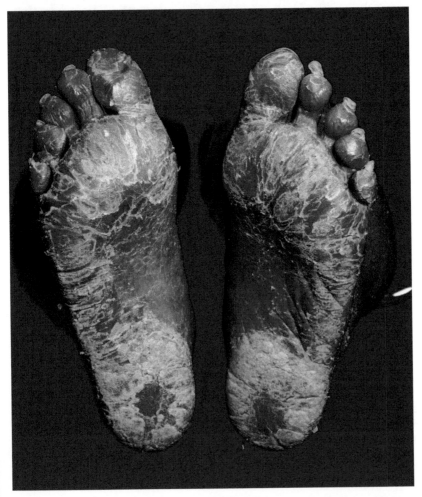

Fig. 4. Plantar keratoderma in a patient with SS.

Fig. 5. Typical nail changes and palmar keratoderma in a patient with SS.

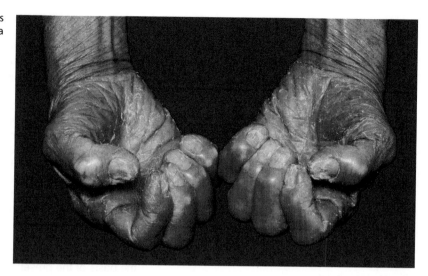

The most commonly noted histopathologic features in SS include the presence of a dermal perivascular to bandlike or interface lymphoid infiltrate at the dermoepidermal junction, with lymphocytic cytologic atypia, accompanying eosinophilia, and reactive epidermal changes, such as mild spongiosis, parakeratosis, and acanthosis.[15] These findings are present in many benign inflammatory dermatoses as well. **Figs. 7–9** demonstrate typical histomorphology of SS lesional skin. Some features, such as Pautrier microabscesses, string of pearls, or epidermotropism, are more characteristically found in MF skin lesions.[1] Historically, clinical observation has suggested SS arises de novo or from preexisting MF or a condition designated pre-SS.[14,15,19] Recent data examining specific lymphocytic subsets and detailed phenotype suggest, however, that MF and SS are actually 2 distinct disease processes characterized by unique T-cell subsets, as opposed to representing a variable expression within a continuum of a single disease, thus challenging the clinical

Fig. 6. Ectropion in a patient with SS. (*Adapted from* Kubica AW, Davis MD, Pittelkow MR. Sézary syndrome. In: Hall JC, Hall BJ, editors. Cutaneous lymphoma: diagnosis and treatment. Shelton (CT): People's Medical Publishing House-USA; 2012. p. 104; with permission.)

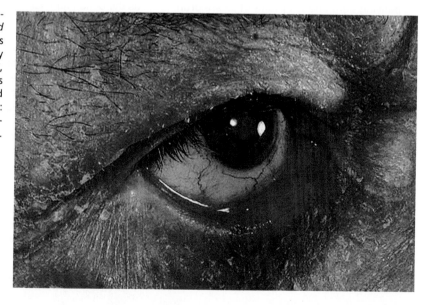

Box 1
Common presenting signs and symptoms of Sézary syndrome

Alopecia
Ectropion

Erythroderma
Exfoliation

Hepatosplenomegaly
Ichthyosis

Leonine facies
Lichenification

Lymphadenopathy
Onychodystrophy

Palmar and plantar keratoderma
Pigmentary changes

Pruritus
Systemic symptoms (fevers, chills, fatigue, weight loss)

Xerosis

Adapted from Kubica AW, Davis MD, Pittelkow MR. Sézary syndrome. In: Hall JC, Hall BJ, editors. Cutaneous lymphoma: diagnosis and treatment. Shelton (CT): People's Medical Publishing House-USA; 2012. p. 104; with permission.

Box 2
Key features of Sézary syndrome

- SS is most common among white men and increases in prevalence with age.

- The required finding on physical examination is erythroderma. The most common accompanying signs and symptoms of SS are pruritus, lymphadenopathy, ectropion, and nail changes.

- The most common histopathologic finding in SS is the presence of an upper dermal band-like and perivascular lymphoid infiltrate with variable cytologic atypia. The histopathologic findings, however, are often nonspecific and similar changes can be observed in many benign conditions. More classic diagnostic features of epidermotropism and Pautrier microabscess formation are infrequently observed.

- Beyond the classic B2 criteria for diagnosis of SS, novel immunochemical and molecular advances have identified potential markers of SS, such as Twist, T-plastin, KIR3DL2, NKp46, CD164, FCRL3, CCR4, CCR7, CCR10, and CD158K. These biomarkers may be incorporated in future diagnostic criteria of SS.

experience where SS seems to arise from prior MF.[20]

The diagnosis of SS has been refined over the decades to its current definition, but its origins trace back to the atypical circulating cells that were first described by Sézary and Bouvrain in 1938.[21] These cells, originally termed *cellules monstreuses*, were observed in the setting of generalized red skin (*l'homme rouge*).[21] The term, *Sézary syndrome*, was eventually coined in 1961 by Taswell and Winkelmann at Mayo Clinic,[22] named after the unique appearance of the Sézary cell, which appears cerebriform by high-power, oil-immersion evaluation of the peripheral blood smear and by electron microscopy. These cells can be appreciated in **Fig. 10**. In the 1970s and 1980s, the diagnosis of SS was established on the basis of the presence of erythroderma as well as definitive hematologic peripheral blood smear abnormalities, defined as the presence of 1000 Sézary cells/mm^3 or greater.[14] This method of quantification has limitations, however, in particular interobserver variability and hematopathologic experience in the interpretation of peripheral blood smear abnormalities.[3,16]

DIAGNOSIS: ANCILLARY STUDIES

With further advances in the understanding of the medical and molecular pathobiology of CTCL, and SS in particular, the diagnosis of SS has undergone periodic revisions by international CTCL consensus committees and has become a more rigorously defined disease entity. As part of these efforts, the ISCL and the EORTC have provided guidelines regarding TNMB staging for CTCL, with the most recent guidelines from 2007 serving as the benchmark for diagnosis.[16,19] These guidelines delineate and differentiate SS from other erythrodermic CTCLs. Specifically, SS is defined as T4 (>80% of total body surface area manifesting erythema) and B2 (high blood tumor burden, defined as molecular evidence of clonality by T-cell gene rearrangement in the blood, absolute Sézary cell count ≥1000/mm^3, CD4/CD8 ratio ≥10 by flow cytometry, and abnormal immunophenotype, including loss of CD7 [≥40%] or CD26 [≥30%]), as detailed in **Table 1**.[16] The difficulties of diagnosing SS are described in **Box 3**.

Recognizing that the main challenge to the diagnosis of SS focuses on the identification of Sézary cells in the blood, various recent studies have taken innovative approaches to attempt to identify these cells more accurately.[23] In addition to the loss of CD7 and CD26, some studies have also correlated the presence of FOXP3$^+$, CD25$^+$ cells within Sézary cells in SS patients. The specificity

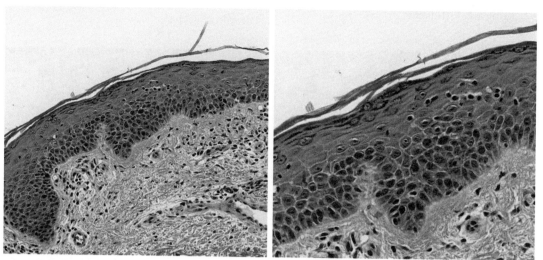

Fig. 7. Occasional atypical lymphocytes present in the epidermis with minimal spongiosis or inflammatory infiltrate (biopsy of erythrodermic skin in a patient with SS; hematoxylin-eosin stain, original magnification ×100 [*left*] and ×200 [*right*]).

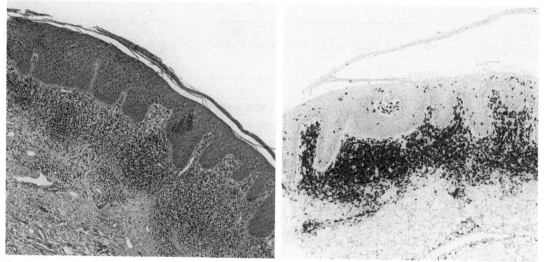

Fig. 8. Upper dermal bandlike infiltrate of atypical CD3+ lymphocytes (biopsy of erythrodermic skin in a patient with SS: hematoxylin-eosin stain, original magnification ×50 [*left*]; CD3 stain, original magnification ×50 [*right*]).

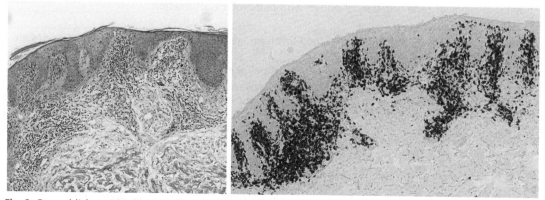

Fig. 9. Dermal lichenoid infiltrate of atypical CD3+ lymphocytes with foci of epidermotropism (biopsy of erythrodermic skin in a patient with SS: hematoxylin-eosin stain, original magnification ×50 [*left*]; CD3 stain, original magnification ×50 [*right*]).

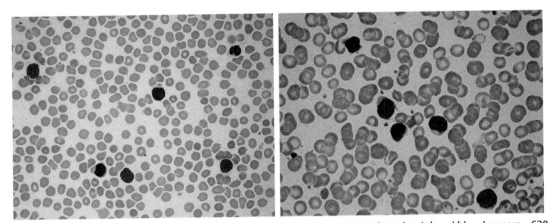

Fig. 10. Large atypical lymphocytes, or Sézary cells, are seen, with scant cytoplasm (peripheral blood smears ×630 [*left*] and ×1000 [*right*]). (*Adapted from* Kubica AW, Davis MD, Pittelkow MR. Sézary syndrome. In: Hall JC, Hall BJ, editors. Cutaneous lymphoma: diagnosis and treatment. Shelton (CT): People's Medical Publishing House-USA; 2012. p. 106; with permission.)

Table 1
TNMB staging for MF and SS, based on 2007 ISCL/EORTC criteria

Stage	Criteria
T: tumor stage	
T1	Patches, papules, and/or plaques <10% body surface area
T2	Patches, plaques ≥10% body surface area
T3	One or more tumors (≥1 cm in diameter)
T4[a]	Erythroderma (erythema ≥80% of body surface area)
N: nodal stage	
N0	No clinically abnormal peripheral LNs
N1[b]	Clinically abnormal peripheral LNs, histopathology Dutch grade 2 or NCI LN0–2
N2[b]	Clinically abnormal peripheral LNs, histopathology Dutch grade 2 or NCI LN3
N3	Clinically abnormal peripheral LNs, histopathology Dutch grade 3–4 or NCI LN4; clone positive or negative
Nx	Clinically abnormal peripheral LNs, no histopathology provided
M: Metastases, visceral involvement	
M0	No visceral organ involvement
M1	Visceral organ involvement with pathologic confirmation
B: peripheral blood stage	
B0[b]	Absence of significant blood involvement: ≤5% of peripheral blood lymphocytes are Sézary cells
B1[b]	Low blood tumor burden: >5% of peripheral blood lymphocytes are Sézary cells
B2[a]	High blood tumor burden: requires positive clonal rearrangement of TCR PLUS one of the following: absolute Sézary cell count ≥1000/mm^3; expanded CD4$^+$ or CD3$^+$ cells with CD4/CD8 ratio ≥10; expanded CD4$^+$ cells with abnormal immunophenotype, including loss of CD7 (≥40%) or CD26 (≥30%)

Abbreviations: LN, lymph node; NCI, National Cancer Institute.
[a] Necessary criteria for SS.
[b] Can be divided into stages a (clone negative) and b (clone positive) if information on clone via polymerase chain reaction or Southern blot analysis of TCR is available.
Adapted from Olsen E, Vonderheid E, Pimpinelli N, et al, ISCL/EORTC. Revisions to the staging and classification of mycosis fungoides and Sézary syndrome: a proposal of the International Society for Cutaneous Lymphomas (ISCL) and the cutaneous lymphoma task force of the European Organization of Research and Treatment of Cancer (EORTC). Blood 2007;110:1715; with permission.

Box 3
Pitfalls in diagnosis of Sézary syndrome

- Only approximately 60% of skin biopsies are diagnostic of CTCL where the diagnosis of SS is eventually established. Lesional skin of MF is more frequently diagnostic than skin biopsy of SS.

- Recent studies have identified MF and SS as 2 distinct disease entities based on immunophenotyping of T-cell subsets rather than a spectrum within the same malignant T-cell clonal process, as previously thought. Specifically, MF arises from resident effector memory T cells, and SS arises from central memory T cells.

- For erythrodermic patients, evaluation for systemic symptoms is key, as is evaluation of peripheral blood for flow cytometry, presence of Sézary cells, and identification of a clonal T-cell gene rearrangement. Evidence of leukemic involvement following B2 criteria is crucial for SS diagnosis.

- It is important to differentiate SS from other types of erythrodermic CTCL, including MF with a separate leukemic disorder and erythrodermic MF. Although some studies have reported SS arising from preexisting MF, this is rare and likely represents a distinct disease process.

- Diagnosis of SS is based on the leukemic, hematologic criteria, defined as molecular evidence of clonality by T-cell gene rearrangement in the blood, absolute Sézary cell count $\geq 1000/mm^3$, CD4/CD8 ratio ≥ 10 by flow cytometry, and abnormal immunophenotype, including loss of CD7 ($\geq 40\%$) or CD26 ($\geq 30\%$).

T-cell antigen receptor, TCR-Vβ, and CD158K allowed for specific identification of all SS cases.[23]

More recently, whole peripheral blood gene expression analysis has identified increased expression of certain markers in SS patients.[29] Much of the focus of this research has been on T-plastin (PLS3) and the transcription factor Twist.[29] In a study of 81 SS patients, gene expression profiling was conducted by quantitative polymerase chain reaction analysis for PLS3, Twist, killer cell immunoglobulin-like receptor 3DL2 (KIR3DL2), and natural killer cell p46-related protein (NKp46), and these markers were found to be highly sensitive for diagnosis of SS. Twist was the most sensitive, with a 91% positivity amongst the SS patients.[29] Other studies have confirmed these results, with PLS3 and Twist up-regulation identified in the malignant T-cell population of SS patients.[25,30–33] Additionally, PLS3 can serve to differentiate MF from SS, because this biomarker is present in higher quantities in SS than MF patients, unaffected subjects, and inflammatory controls.[25,30,31] Such studies that differentiate MF and SS reinforce the recent findings of Campbell and colleagues[20] that SS and MF arise from distinct subsets of T cells: MF arises from effector memory T cells whereas SS is proposed as a malignancy of central memory T cells. Considering these advances, there is an urgent need for further investigation and cooperative studies by the United States Cutaneous Lymphoma Consortium, EORTC, and ISCL to evaluate and validate specific, reliable, affordable, widely available and accessible diagnostic criteria for CTCL and SS specifically. Such studies would assist with standardization of the diagnosis worldwide and allow for prompt identification, early treatment, and accurate monitoring of clinical progression in the future of this aggressive malignancy.

DIFFERENTIAL DIAGNOSIS

When attempting to differentiate SS from other dermatologic entities, important conditions within the differential diagnosis manifest erythroderma, which is the central and defining physical finding of SS, as well as conditions with circulating Sézary cell–like cells. **Table 2** summarizes conditions, both benign and neoplastic, that are commonly considered in the differential diagnosis of SS. Most frequently, these include generalized atopic dermatitis, irritant or allergic contact dermatitis, parapsoriasis, pityriasis rubra pilaris, and erythrodermic hypersensitivity reactions to various medications.[15]

Additionally, less common variants of CTCL are among the uncommon to rare conditions that

of this subset remains unclear, however, considering discrepancies reported in *in vivo* studies.[1,23] Recently, the authors have also identified this T-regulatory (Treg)–like population among SS patients, but on testing their functional status, Sézary cells failed to perform as Treg in specific assays.[24] Chemokine receptors, such as CCR4, CCR7, and CCR10, have also been studied in relation to circulating CLA+, CD4+ T cells of SS that play a presumed role in the skin homing of these malignant T cells.[1,20,25,26] These chemokine receptors may be closely linked pathogenically and used to identify Sézary cells.[23] Anti–T-cell receptor (TCR)-Vβ chain expression, CD158K, CD164, and FCRL3 have also been identified as markers in SS diagnosis.[23,27,28] In a study of 17 SS patients, however, no one test was found able to diagnose all patients with SS, but combining flow cytometry gating on a

Table 2 Differential diagnosis of Sézary syndrome	
Benign	
Atopic dermatitis	Lupus erythematosus
Bullous pemphigoid	Parapsoriasis
Contact dermatitis	Pityriasis rubra pilaris
Cutaneous drug reaction	Psoriasis
Dermal reticulosis	Purpura
Dermatomyositis	Sarcoidosis
DRESS syndrome	Seborrheic dermatitis
Generalized anaphylaxis	Urticaria
Graft-versus-host disease	
Malignant	
Acute or chronic leukemia	Erythrodermic MF
CTCL spectrum disease	Pre-SS

Abbreviation: DRESS, drug reaction with eosinophilia and systemic symptoms.

Adapted from Kubica AW, Davis MD, Pittelkow MR. Sézary syndrome. In: Hall JC, Hall BJ, editors. Cutaneous lymphoma: diagnosis and treatment. Shelton (CT): People's Medical Publishing House-USA; 2012. p. 108; with permission.

exhibit erythroderma in the differential diagnosis. As a unifying diagnosis and terminology developed at a time when the T lymphocyte was first identified by phenotypic markers and applied to MF and SS, CTCL was thought to represent a spectrum of disease, with SS the more aggressive, advanced, and severe form.[16,17] **Table 3**, following recommendations from the ISCL, illustrates the categorization of erythrodermic CTCL based on preceding MF and degree of leukemic involvement, with primary, or de novo, SS having no prior MF.[19] In various studies, SS has been considered to evolve from previous pre-SS states or in

patients with previously diagnosed MF.[6,15,19,34] These clinical presentations need to be reconciled, however, with more recent detailed phenotypic findings demonstrating that MF and leukemic variants of CTCL, such as SS, are most likely distinct disease processes.[20] Studies show that the pathogenesis of SS is related to malignant clonal expansion of a central memory T-cell population, whereas MF is a malignant, clonal lymphoproliferative disorder of effector memory T cells.[20]

The diagnosis of SS is based on assimilating the clinical history and physical examination, appropriate hematologic studies of flow cytometry, and molecular studies and supportive pathologic findings on skin biopsy as well as lymph node and bone marrow, as determined by the initial staging evaluation. In the diagnosis of SS, it is paramount to incorporate the full clinical presentation and pathologic findings. Ultimately, the main distinguishing factor that differentiates SS from the other conditions included in the differential diagnosis is the presence of and extent of blood involvement, as currently defined by the EORTC and ISCL.[16,19]

PROGNOSIS

Current medical data from various institutions, both in the United States and internationally, have consistently reported a generally poor prognosis for SS. The survival and prognostic data for SS in particular, however, are difficult to establish at times, given the continually evolving understanding of CTCL and the relative rarity of SS compared with other subtypes of CTCL. As a result of homogenization of CTCL reporting at several clinical centers, studies including SS have typically combined this disease entity with more indolent forms of CTCL, such as MF, thus creating limitations in assessing actual survival, progression, and outcomes of SS.[3]

Table 3 Variants of CTCL in the differential diagnosis of Sézary syndrome				
CTCL Subtype	**Erythroderma Present**	**Preexisting MF**	**Blood Findings**	**TNMB Designation**
SS	Yes	Rarely	Leukemic	T4 N0–3 M0–1 B2
Erythrodermic MF	Yes	Typically	Absent or minimal	T4 N0–3 M0–1 B0–1
Erythrodermic CTCL NOS	Yes	Absent	Absent or minimal	T4 N0–3 M0–1 B0–1
MF with leukemic findings, nonerythrodermic SS	No	Typically	Leukemic	T1–3 N0–3 M0–1 B2

Abbreviation: NOS, not otherwise specified.

Adapted from Vonderheid EC, Bernengo MG, Burg G, et al, ISCL. Update on erythrodermic cutaneous T-cell lymphoma: report of the International Society for Cutaneous Lymphomas. J Am Acad Dermatol 2002;46:96; with permission.

The 2 largest survival studies of SS patients in the recent literature derive from large clinical experiences reported by Mayo Clinic and MD Anderson Cancer Center.[6,35] The Mayo Clinic experience, with a cohort of 176 SS patients, found a median survival of 4.0 years from time of diagnosis.[6] Similarly, the MD Anderson experience of 184 SS patients found a median overall survival of 4.98 years.[35] Among other studies of CTCL that specified data for SS patients, the median survival was 2.5 to 4 years.[7–10,13,36,37] When involvement of the viscera was identified, median survival has been 2.5 years or less.[11,13,37] Beyond visceral involvement, numerous prognostic factors associated with worse outcomes have been outlined in CTCL and SS studies, including advanced age, increased leukemic burden in the blood, increased lactic dehydrogenase levels, enlargement of peripheral lymph nodes, low percentage of CD8[+] cells in lymph nodes, large cell transformation, prior MF, loss of interleukin 16, loss of CDKN2A-CDKN2B, and elevated white blood cell count.[2,6,10,35,38–40] In an effort to provide further guidelines for prognosis and survival, Olsen and colleagues,[41] in collaboration with the ISCL, published new recommendations for standardization of clinical assessment and endpoints in CTCL patients to provide more uniform and consistent criteria for international investigations of CTCL. Additionally, the use of the CTCL severity index could assist with estimation of prognosis in SS patients.[42]

While diagnosis remains a challenge in many situations, the pathophysiology and definition of SS has undergone significant evolution over the last several decades. Continued pursuits are ongoing to develop a better understanding of the molecular and clinical behavior of this multifaceted and complex malignancy.

REFERENCES

1. Hwang ST, Janik JE, Jaffe ES, et al. Mycosis fungoides and Sézary syndrome. Lancet 2008;371: 945–57.

2. Kim EJ, Lin J, Junkins-Hopkins JM, et al. Mycosis fungoides and Sézary syndrome: an update. Curr Oncol Rep 2006;8:376–86.

3. Olsen EA, Rook AH, Zic J, et al. Sézary syndrome: immunopathogenesis, literature review of therapeutic options, and recommendations for therapy by the United States Cutaneous Lymphoma Consortium (USCLC). J Am Acad Dermatol 2011;64: 352–404.

4. Criscione VD, Weinstock MA. Incidence of cutaneous T-cell lymphoma in the United States, 1973-2002. Arch Dermatol 2007;143:854–9.

5. Bradford PT, Devesa SS, Anderson WF, et al. Cutaneous lymphoma incidence patterns in the United States: a population-based study of 3884 cases. Blood 2009;113:5064–73.

6. Kubica AW, Davis MD, Weaver AL, et al. Sézary syndrome: a study of 176 patients at Mayo Clinic. J Am Acad Dermatol 2012;67:1189–99.

7. Bernengo MG, Quaglino P, Novelli M, et al. Prognostic factors in Sézary syndrome: a multivariate analysis of clinical, haematological and immunological features. Ann Oncol 1998;9:857–63.

8. Foulc P, N'Guyen JM, Dreno B. Prognostic factors in Sézary syndrome: a study of 28 patients. Br J Dermatol 2003;149:1152–8.

9. Vidulich KA, Talpur R, Bassett RL, et al. Overall survival in erythrodermic cutaneous T-cell lymphoma: an analysis of prognostic factors in a cohort of patients with erythrodermic cutaneous T-cell lymphoma. Int J Dermatol 2009;48:243–52.

10. Agar NS, Wedgeworth E, Crichton S, et al. Survival outcomes and prognostic factors in mycosis fungoides/Sézary syndrome: validation of the revised International Society for Cutaneous Lymphomas/European Organisation for Research and Treatment of Cancer staging proposal. J Clin Oncol 2010;28: 4730–9.

11. Zackheim HS, Amin S, Kashani-Sabet M, et al. Prognosis in cutaneous T-cell lymphoma by skin stage: long-term survival in 489 patients. J Am Acad Dermatol 1999;40:418–25.

12. Booken N, Nicolay JP, Weiss C, et al. Cutaneous tumor cell load correlates with survival in patients with Sézary syndrome. J Dtsch Dermatol Ges 2013;11: 67–79.

13. Diamandidou E, Colome M, Fayad L, et al. Prognostic factor analysis in mycosis fungoides/Sézary syndrome. J Am Acad Dermatol 1999;40(6 Pt 1): 914–24.

14. Buechner SA, Winkelmann RK. Sézary syndrome: a clinicopathologic study of 39 cases. Arch Dermatol 1983;119:979–86.

15. Diwan AH, Prieto VG, Herling M, et al. Primary Sézary syndrome commonly shows low-grade cytologic atypia and an absence of epidermotropism. Am J Clin Pathol 2005;123:510–5.

16. Olsen E, Vonderheid E, Pimpinelli N, et al, ISCL/EORTC. Revisions to the staging and classification of mycosis fungoides and Sézary syndrome: a proposal of the International Society for Cutaneous Lymphomas (ISCL) and the cutaneous lymphoma task force of the European Organization of Research and Treatment of Cancer (EORTC). Blood 2007;110: 1713–22.

17. Vonderheid EC, Zhang Q, Lessin SR, et al. Use of serum soluble interleukin-2 receptor levels to monitor the progression of cutaneous T-cell lymphoma. J Am Acad Dermatol 1998;38(2 Pt 1):207–20.

18. Olerud JE, Kulin PA, Chew DE, et al. Cutaneous T-cell lymphoma: evaluation of pretreatment skin biopsy specimens by a panel of pathologists. Arch Dermatol 1992;128:501–7.

19. Vonderheid EC, Bernengo MG, Burg G, et al, ISCL. Update on erythrodermic cutaneous T-cell lymphoma: report of the International Society for Cutaneous Lymphomas. J Am Acad Dermatol 2002;46: 95–106.

20. Campbell JJ, Clark RA, Watanabe R, et al. Sézary syndrome and mycosis fungoides arise from distinct T-cell subsets: a biologic rationale for their distinct clinical behaviors. Blood 2010;116:767–71.

21. Sézary A, Bouvrain Y. Erythrodermie avec présence des cellules monstrueuses dans le dermeet le sang circulant. Bull Soc Fr Dermatol Syphiligr 1938;45: 254–60.

22. Taswell HF, Winkelmann RK. Sézary syndrome: a malignant reticulemic erythroderma. JAMA 1961; 177:465–72.

23. Klemke CD, Brade J, Weckesser S, et al. The diagnosis of Sézary syndrome on peripheral blood by flow cytometry requires the use of multiple markers. Br J Dermatol 2008;159:871–80.

24. Wada DA, Pittelkow MR, Comfere NI, et al. CD4(+) CD25(+)FOXP3(+) malignant T cells in Sézary syndrome are not necessarily functional regulatory T cells. J Am Acad Dermatol 2013;69:485–9.

25. Begue E, Jean-Louis F, Bagot M, et al. Inducible expression and pathophysiologic functions of T-plastin in cutaneous T-cell lymphoma. Blood 2012;120:143–54.

26. Sokolowska-Wojdylo M, Wenzel J, Gaffal E, et al. Absence of CD26 expression on skin-homing CLA+ CD4+ T lymphocytes in peripheral blood is a highly sensitive marker for early diagnosis and therapeutic monitoring of patients with Sézary syndrome. Clin Exp Dermatol 2005;30:702–6.

27. Morice WG, Katzmann JA, Pittelkow MR, et al. A comparison of morphologic features, flow cytometry, TCR-Vbeta analysis, and TCR-PCR in qualitative and quantitative assessment of peripheral blood involvement by Sézary syndrome. Am J Clin Pathol 2006;125:364–74.

28. Wysocka M, Kossenkov AV, Benoit BM, et al. CD164 and FCRL3 are highly expressed on CD4+CD26− T cells in Sézary syndrome patients. J Invest Dermatol 2014;134(1):229–36.

29. Michel L, Jean-Louis F, Begue E, et al. Use of PLS3, Twist, CD158k/KIR3DL2, and NKp46 gene expression combination for reliable Sézary syndrome diagnosis. Blood 2013;121:1477–8.

30. Tang N, Gibson H, Germeroth T, et al. T-plastin (PLS3) gene expression differentiates Sézary syndrome from mycosis fungoides and inflammatory skin diseases and can serve as a biomarker to monitor disease progression. Br J Dermatol 2010; 162:463–6.

31. Goswami M, Duvic M, Dougherty A, et al. Increased Twist expression in advanced stage of mycosis fungoides and Sézary syndrome. J Cutan Pathol 2012; 39:500–7.

32. vanDoorn R, Dijkman R, Vermeer MH, et al. Aberrant expression of the tyrosine kinase receptor EphA4 and the transcription factor twist in Sézary syndrome identified by gene expression analysis. Cancer Res 2004;64:5578–86.

33. Su MW, Dorocicz I, Dragowska WH, et al. Aberrant expression of T-plastin in Sezary cells. Cancer Res 2003;63:7122–7.

34. Buechner SA, Winkelmann RK. Pre-Sézary erythroderma evolving to Sézary syndrome: a report of seven cases. Arch Dermatol 1983;119:285–91.

35. Talpur R, Singh L, Daulat S, et al. Long-term outcomes of 1,263 patients with mycosis fungoides and Sézary syndrome from 1982 to 2009. Clin Cancer Res 2012;18:5051–60.

36. Willemze R, Jaffe ES, Burg G, et al. WHO-EORTC classification for cutaneous lymphomas. Blood 2005;105:3768–85.

37. Kim YH, Liu HL, Mraz-Gernhard S, et al. Long-term outcome of 525 patients with mycosis fungoides and Sézary syndrome: clinical prognostic factors and risk for disease progression. Arch Dermatol 2003;139:857–66.

38. Richmond J, Tuzova M, Parks A, et al. Interleukin-16 as a marker of Sézary syndrome onset and stage. J Clin Immunol 2011;31:39–50.

39. Laharanne E, Chevret E, Idrissi Y, et al. CDKN2A-CDKN2B deletion defines an aggressive subset of cutaneous T-cell lymphoma. Mod Pathol 2010;23: 547–58.

40. Vonderheid EC, Pena J, Nowell P. Sézary cell counts in erythrodermic cutaneous T-cell lymphoma: implications for prognosis and staging. Leuk Lymphoma 2006;47:1841–56.

41. Olsen EA, Whittaker S, Kim YH, et al, International Society for Cutaneous Lymphomas, United States Cutaneous Lymphoma Consortium, Cutaneous Lymphoma Task Force of the European Organisation for Research and Treatment of Cancer. Clinical end points and response criteria in mycosis fungoides and Sézary syndrome: a consensus statement of the International Society for Cutaneous Lymphomas, the United States Cutaneous Lymphoma Consortium, and the Cutaneous Lymphoma Task Force of the European Organisation for Research and Treatment of Cancer. J Clin Oncol 2011;29:2598–607.

42. Klemke CD, Mansmann U, Poenitz N, et al. Prognostic factors and prediction of prognosis by the CTCL Severity Index in mycosis fungoides and Sézary syndrome. Br J Dermatol 2005;153:118–24.

Cutaneous CD30-Positive Lymphoproliferative Disorders

Werner Kempf, MD[a,b],*

KEYWORDS

- Lymphoma • Cutaneous • CD30 • Lymphomatoid papulosis • Anaplastic large-cell lymphoma
- Borderline • Clinico-pathological correlation • Systemic

KEY POINTS

- Lymphomatoid papulosis (LyP), primary cutaneous anaplastic large-cell lymphoma (pcALCL), and borderline lesions constitute the group of cutaneous CD30+ lymphoproliferative disorders (CD30+ LPDs). These diseases manifest with a broad histologic and phenotypic spectrum.
- The overlapping histopathological features of LyP and pcALCL with themselves and with other cutaneous and systemic lymphomas underscore the importance of careful correlation with clinical findings and staging results.
- CD30 is not only a diagnostic marker for CD30+ LPDs, but its expression is of prognostic impact in other lymphomas. In addition, anti-CD30 antibody-based therapeutic strategies target tumor cells in CD30+ LPDs and other lymphomas.

ABSTRACT

Cutaneous CD30+ lymphoproliferative disorders are the second most common types of cutaneous T-cell lymphomas. They represent a well-defined spectrum encompassing lymphomatoid papulosis (LyP), primary cutaneous anaplastic large-cell lymphoma (pcALCL), and borderline lesions. They share the expression of CD30 as a common phenotypic hallmark, but they differ in their clinical presentation, course, and histologic features. New variants have been recently identified, including CD8+ epidermotropic LyP type D, angioinvasive LyP type E, and ALK-positive pcALCL. This review describes clinical, histopathologic, and phenotypic variants; their differential diagnoses (benign and malignant); and the role of CD30 as a diagnostic, prognostic, and therapeutic marker.

OVERVIEW

Primary cutaneous CD30+ lymphoproliferative disorders (CD30+ LPDs) are the second most common form of cutaneous T-cell lymphomas (CTCLs) and account for approximately 30% of all primary cutaneous lymphomas (CLs).[1,2] CD30+ LPDs represent a spectrum of disorders encompassing lymphomatoid papulosis (LyP), primary cutaneous anaplastic large-cell lymphoma (pcALCL), and so-called borderline lesions. Their common phenotypic hallmark is the expression of CD30 by atypical lymphocytes. CD30, which was discovered in 1982 by H. Stein and coworkers in Berlin and was initially referred to as Ki-1,[3] is a cytokine receptor belonging to the tumor necrosis factor receptor superfamily. It is engaged in the control of tumor cell growth with divergent effects on apoptosis and

Disclosure Statement: The author has no conflicts of interest and no source of funding in the article to declare.
[a] Kempf und Pfaltz, Histologische Diagnostik, Seminarstrasse 1, Zürich CH-8042, Switzerland; [b] Department of Dermatology, University Hospital, Zürich CH-8091, Switzerland.
* Kempf und Pfaltz, Histologische Diagnostik, Seminarstrasse 1, Zürich CH-8042, Switzerland.
E-mail address: kempf@kempf-pfaltz.ch

Surgical Pathology 7 (2014) 203–228
http://dx.doi.org/10.1016/j.path.2014.02.001
1875-9181/14/$ – see front matter © 2014 Elsevier Inc. All rights reserved.

proliferation in cutaneous CD30+ LPDs and systemic CD30+ lymphomas.[4,5]

LyP and pcALCL show overlapping histomorphological and phenotypic features, but they significantly differ in their clinical presentation. Moreover, CD30+ LPDs show overlapping or even identical histomorphological and phenotypic features with secondary cutaneous involvement by systemic CD30+ lymphomas. This implies that careful clinico-pathologic correlation and staging are mandatory elements in the diagnostic workup of cutaneous infiltrates of CD30+ atypical lymphocytes.[6,7] Both LyP and pcALCL exhibit a wide spectrum of clinical, histologic, and phenotypic variants. In addition, expression of CD30 can be seen in variable degree in other CLs and in systemic lymphomas. In addition, the presence of large CD30+ cells is not restricted to lymphomas, as various inflammatory and infectious diseases can harbor CD30+ medium-sized to large atypical-appearing T-cells, thereby simulating CD30+ LPDs and representing diagnostic pitfalls.[8,9] As a consequence, the diagnosis of CD30+ LPD has to be based on the correlation of clinical, histopathologic, phenotypic, and genetic features, as well as staging results. In contrast to systemic ALCL (sALCL) and Hodgkin lymphoma (HL), cutaneous CD30+ LPDs exhibit a markedly favorable prognosis.[6] To emphasize these biologic differences between primary cutaneous and systemic CD30+ lymphomas, cutaneous CD30+ LPDs are listed as distinct nosologic entities in the current World Health Organization (WHO) classification (4th edition, 2008).[10]

As a consequence of the different course and prognosis between cutaneous CD30+ LPD and systemic CD30+ lymphomas, the therapeutic approach to CD30+ LPD differs from the treatment modalities used in systemic CD30+ lymphomas.[7] Recently, CD30 has become a therapeutic target for antibody-based therapy. Remarkably, the expression of CD30 assessed by immunohistochemistry does not appear to correlate directly with efficacy of anti-CD30 antibody-based drugs, leaving open the question of how to assess CD30 as a therapeutic marker in the various forms of CTCL and other lymphomas.[11] In addition, an increasing number of studies have demonstrated the value of CD30 as a prognostic marker in other lymphomas, such as mycosis fungoides (MF), as the expression of CD30 by dermal lymphocytes in patch and plaque stage is associated with impaired prognosis.[12]

Several characteristics of cutaneous CD30+ LPD, such as the discrepancy between the pleomorphic and anaplastic cytomorphology of the tumor cells being suggestive of a high grade malignancy and the paradoxic biologic behavior with a favorable prognosis and the spontaneous regression of lesions in LyP, render CD30+ LPD an interesting model for lymphomagenesis.

This review article summarizes the clinicopathologic features of CD30+ LPDs, including recently identified new variants, their differential diagnoses, and the role of CD30 as a prognostic marker and therapeutic target in various types of CTCLs.

LYP

OVERVIEW

LyP was first described by the dermatologist Warren L. Macaulay, MD, as a chronic recurrent, self-healing papulo-nodular skin eruption with histologic features of a malignant lymphoma.[13,14] Since the first description of the disease, there is a debate about whether LyP is merely a benign lymphoproliferative disorder or whether it should be regarded as a low-grade malignant lymphoma. The excellent prognosis and the lack of mortality would justify the concept of a benign lymphoproliferation. On the other hand, the association with clonally related cutaneous and systemic lymphomas and the morphologic and phenotypic similarities with pcALCL may argue for LyP as an indolent lymphoma that is tightly controlled by the host immune response or intrinsic growth factors.

DIAGNOSIS: CLINICAL FEATURES

LyP presents with grouped or disseminated papules and smaller nodules that evolve and spontaneously regress within a few weeks. Sometimes ulceration precedes regression and hypopigmented or hyperpigmented varioliform scars may be left behind after regression of the lesions (Fig. 1). The number of lesions in LyP can vary from a few to hundreds of lesions. The disease duration is highly variable and ranges from several weeks to years or even decades. LyP mostly affects adults, but can develop in children as well.[15,16] Unusual clinical variants of LyP include acral and other regional forms of LyP, with lesions limited to one body region.[17] Follicular LyP may present with pustular lesions simulating folliculitis.[18,19] Papular, self-regressing lesions overlapping with localized MF-like patches may be referred to as persistent agmination of LyP (PALP). Some investigators consider this form a variant of localized LyP with the potential to involve other skin regions, whereas others regard PALP as a composite lymphoma (for review see Ref.[20]). Another matter of debate is the issue of oral

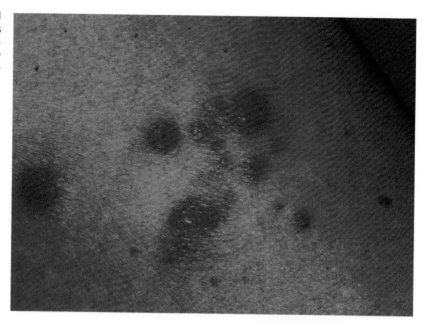

Fig. 1. LyP: grouped papulo-nodular lesions on the arm. The individual lesions spontaneously regress within a few weeks.

mucosal involvement in LyP, which is uncommon, and its relationship to traumatic ulcerative granuloma with stromal eosinophilia, which contains CD30+ large atypical lymphoid cells, a clonal T-cell population in a subset of cases, and shows an excellent prognosis.[21,22]

DIAGNOSIS: MICROSCOPIC FEATURES

Five histologic subtypes (A–E) have been delineated (Table 1). These histologic types can be concurrently present in an individual patient.[23] The histologic features of LyP types A to C were previously described in detail.[23] Briefly, LyP type A is the most common histologic manifestation, accounting for 75% of all LyP specimens.[6,23] It shows a wedge-shaped dermal infiltrate of medium-sized to large pleomorphic and anaplastic lymphoid cells in the background of numerous inflammatory cells, including neutrophils, eosinophils, and histiocytes (Fig. 2). LyP type B is characterized by an epidermotropic infiltrate of mostly small to medium-sized lymphocytes with cerebriform nuclei, thereby resembling histologic features of MF or Sézary syndrome (Fig. 3). LyP type C displays a nodular cohesive infiltrate of large atypical lymphoid cells and only a few intermingled reactive inflammatory cells (Fig. 4). The LyP types D and E have been recently described.[24,25] Type D shows epidermotropic infiltrates of CD8+ (100%) and CD30+ (90%) atypical, mostly small to medium-sized pleomorphic lymphocytes, thereby differing from LyP type B, which carries a CD4+ T-helper phenotype and displays variable expression of CD30 (Fig. 5).[24] In addition to the epidermotropic infiltrate, a deep dermal perivascular component may be present in LyP type D. Due to the prominent epidermotropism and its phenotype, LyP type D mimics primary cutaneous aggressive epidermotropic CD8+ cytotoxic T-cell lymphoma.[24,26,27] The angioinvasive LyP type E shows angiocentric and angiodestructive infiltrates of mostly medium-sized atypical lymphocytes with pleomorphic, moderately chromatin-dense nuclei (Fig. 6).[25,28] The infiltration of vascular walls results in destruction of vessels and obliteration by thrombi. As a consequence of vascular damage, extensive hemorrhage, necrosis, and ulceration are found. Because deep dermal and subcutaneous vessels are destroyed, clinically the rapidly evolving, eschar-like necrotic lesions may reach a diameter up to 4 cm and are often larger than the papular-nodular lesions commonly found in LyP (Fig. 7). The additional presence of a few papular lesions and the clinical course with spontaneous regression of the ulcers within weeks followed by recurrences allows its classification in the LyP spectrum. The atypical lymphocytes in LyP type E express CD3, CD8 (70%) or CD4, CD30 (100%), TIA-1, and granzyme B.

One intention to introduce the new histologic types D and E was to make pathologists and dermatopathologists aware of these unusual clinical and histologic manifestations, thereby reducing the risk for misinterpretation of these LyP types as aggressive lymphomas.

Additional rare and unusual histopathological variants of LyP include follicular, syringotropic,

Table 1
LyP: histologic types and differential diagnosis

LyP Type	Histology	Differential Diagnosis	Distinguishing Criteria
Type A	Wedge-shaped infiltrate. Scattered and small clusters of large CD30+ lymphocytes with nuclear pleomorphism and mitotic activity. Numerous histiocytes, eosinophils, neutrophils.	HL MF (transformation)	Staging results (in nodal HL) Patches and plaques in MF vs self-regressing papulonodular lesions in LyP
Type B	Epidermotropic infiltrate of small to medium-sized lymphocytes with atypical, chromatin-dense nuclei and variable expression of CD30 (0%–77%).	MF (patch/plaque stage)	Patches and plaques in MF vs self-regressing papulonodular lesions in LyP
Type C	Nodular cohesive infiltrate of large CD30+ pleomorphic or anaplastic lymphocytes with abundant cytoplasm and mitotic activity. Admixture of only a few eosinophils and neutrophils.	Anaplastic large-cell lymphoma (primary cutaneous or systemic form) MF (large cell transformation) Peripheral T-cell lymphoma, NOS (primary cutaneous or nodal) Adult T-cell leukemia/lymphoma	Clinical presentation with solitary or grouped nodules in pcALCL. Staging results in sALCL. Patches and plaques preceding tumors in MF Lack of CD30 or expression by only a minority of tumor cells. Staging results (nodal) Integration of HTLV-1 in tumor cell genome.
Type D	Epidermotropism of atypical small to medium-sized pleomorphic lymphocytes with expression of CD8 and CD30. Deep dermal or subcutaneous perivascular infiltrates may be present.	PR Primary cutaneous aggressive epidermotropic CD8+ cytotoxic T-cell lymphoma Cutaneous gamma/delta T-cell lymphoma	Unilesional erythematous scaling lesion in PR. Multiple rapidly evolving plaques and nodules with erosions and necrosis. Lack of CD30 expression Multiple plaques with erosions IHC: Expression of TCR gamma
Type E	Angioinvasive, ie, angiocentric and angiodestructive infiltrates of mostly small to medium-sized pleomorphic CD30+ lymphocytes and expression of CD8+ in 70% of the cases. Admixture of eosinophils. Vascular occlusion by atypical lymphocytes and/or thrombi, hemorrhage, extensive necrosis and ulceration.	Extranodal NK/T-cell lymphoma, nasal type Cutaneous gamma/delta T-cell lymphoma Anaplastic large-cell lymphoma (primary cutaneous or systemic form) variant with angiocentric and angiodestructive growth	Association with EBV, mostly secondary cutaneous involvement (staging) IHC: Expression of TCR gamma Clinical presentation with solitary or grouped nodules in pcALCL. Staging results in sALCL.

Abbreviations: EBV, Epstein-Barr virus; HL, Hodgkin lymphoma; HTLV-1, human T-cell leukemia virus type 1; IHC, immunohistochemistry; LyP, lymphomatoid papulosis; MF, mycosis fungoides; NK, natural killer; NOS, not otherwise specified; pcALCL, primary cutaneous anaplastic large-cell lymphoma; PR, pagetoid reticulosis; sALCL, systemic anaplastic large-cell lymphoma; TCR, T-cell receptor.

Fig. 2. LyP, type A: Wedge-shaped dermal infiltrate (HE, original magnification ×10) (*A*) of medium-sized to large lymphoid cells with nuclear pleomorphism in the background of neutrophils, eosinophils, and histiocytes (HE, original magnification ×200) (*B*). Expression of CD30 by single and clustered, atypical lymphocytes (*C*) (APAAP, original magnification ×200).

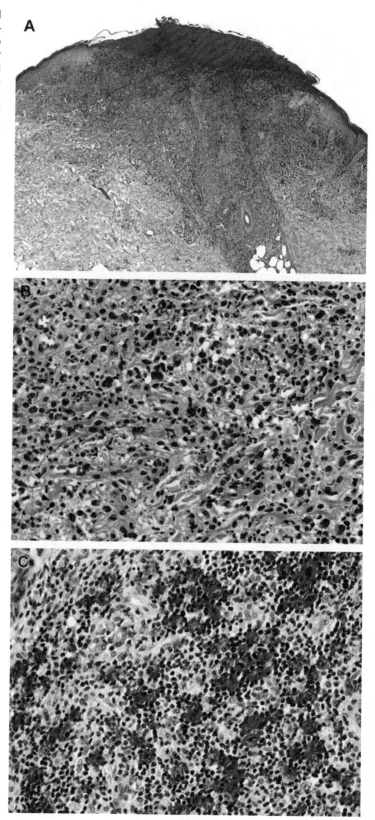

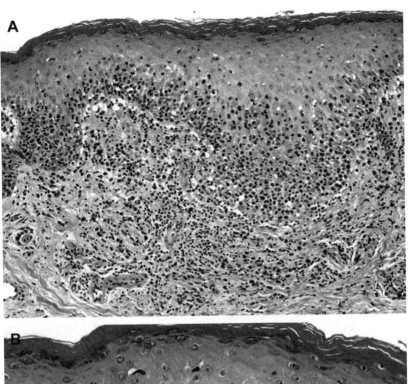

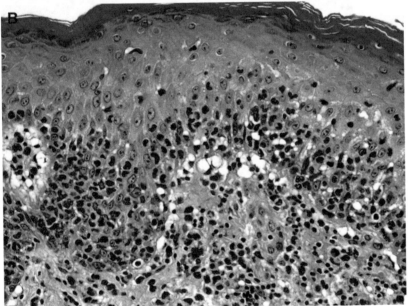

Fig. 3. LyP, type B: Epidermotropic infiltrate (HE, original magnification ×100) (*A*) of small to medium-sized lymphocytes with cerebriform nuclei (*B*) (HE, original magnification ×200).

and granulomatous LyP (reviewed in Ref.[8]). Follicular LyP is associated with predominantly perifollicular infiltrates and folliculotropism of CD30+ atypical lymphocytes.[19,29] Occasionally, follicular mucinosis and collections of neutrophils in the hair follicles are found, the latter giving rise to pustular lesions (pustular LyP).[18,19] Syringotropic LyP shows marked perieccrine infiltrates, which can efface the eccrine units.[30] Noncaseating granulomas are the characteristic feature of granulomatous LyP.[30]

DIAGNOSIS: ANCILLARY STUDIES

The atypical lymphocytes in LyP display the phenotype of activated T-helper cells expressing CD3+, CD4+, CD8−, CD30+, CD45RO+, HLA-DR+, and CD25+. CD30 is consistently expressed by atypical medium-sized to large lymphocytes in all LyP types, except type B, in which variable expression of CD30 (0%–77% of atypical lymphocytes) has been reported in the literature.[23,31] Variable loss of pan T-cell antigens

Fig. 4. LyP, type C: Cohesive dermal infiltrate (HE, original magnification ×10) (*A*) of large atypical lymphoid cells with only a few intermingled reactive inflammatory cells (HE, original magnification ×100) (*B*). Note absence of epidermotropism of tumor cells in this case.

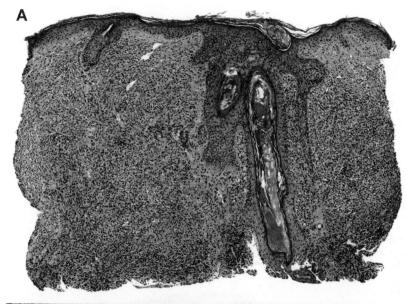

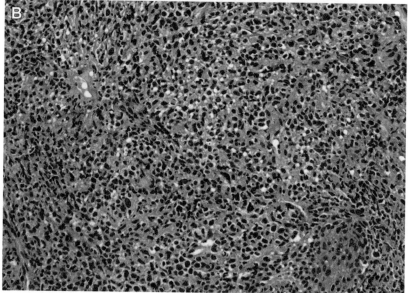

(CD2, CD3, CD5, and/or CD7) can be observed, with CD7 most commonly being absent.[32] A CD4+ and CD45RO+ phenotype is the most common phenotype in LyP, observed in approximately 90% of the cases. However, in the recently described LyP type D (100%) and LyP type E (70%), the atypical lymphocytes usually express a CD8+ phenotype. Furthermore, LyP in children predominantly exhibits a CD8+ phenotype.[33] CD56 expression by atypical CD30+ cells was identified in approximately 10% of LyP cases.[34] Remarkably, expression of cytotoxic molecules, such as TIA-1 and granzyme B, was observed in

most LyP cases.[35] The vast majority of LyP cases express the alpha/beta T-cell receptor (TCR) (beta F1), but expression of the gamma/delta TCR was recently found, particularly in LyP type D.[36,37] Nonetheless, one has to be aware that the course and prognosis of LyP is not influenced by the phenotype of the atypical lymphocytes in LyP.[23,24]

The percentage of detection of monoclonal rearrangement of TCR genes varies from 40% to 100% and may depend on conservation (fresh-frozen vs formalin-fixed paraffin-embedded tissue) and histologic LyP type (ie, number of atypical lymphocytes present in the infiltrate). In our study,

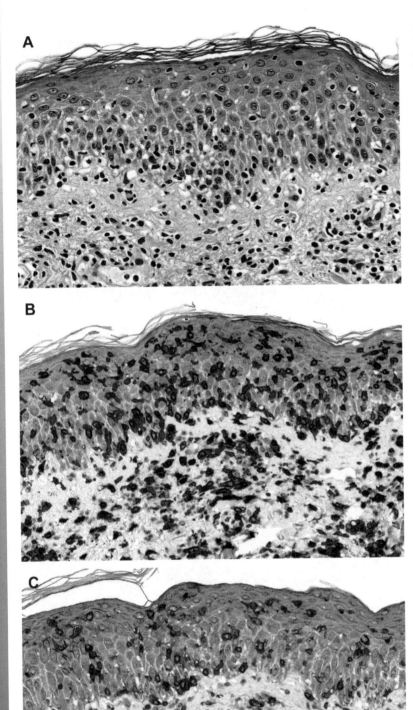

Fig. 5. LyP, type D: Epidermotropic infiltrate (HE, original magnification ×200) (*A*) of small to medium-sized atypical lymphocytes. Expression of CD8 (HE, original magnification ×200) (*B*) and CD30 (*C*) (APAAP, original magnification ×200).

Fig. 6. LyP, type E: Extensive hemorrhage, necrosis, and angiocentric as well as angiodestructive infiltrates (HE, original magnification ×12.5) (*A*) of mostly medium-sized to large atypical lymphocytes with nuclear pleomorphism and admixed eosinophils (*B*) (HE, original magnification ×200).

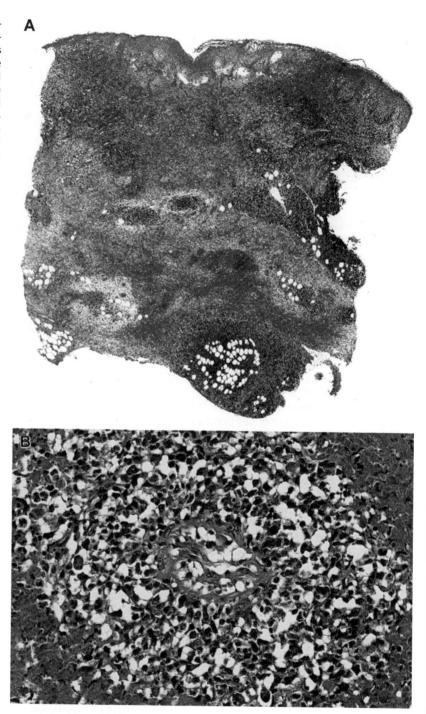

we detected a clonal T-cell population by polymerase chain reaction (PCR) in a minority (22%) of archival LyP specimens. These findings demonstrate that the lack of detection of T-cell clonality does not argue against LyP.[38] The data on the cellular correlate of clonal T cells in LyP derived from microdissection-based studies are highly controversial. One study showed that the CD30+ cells belong to a single T-cell clone, whereas the CD30– lymphocytes were polyclonal in all instances and unrelated to the CD30+ cell clone.[39] Their data indicate that LyP unequivocally represents a monoclonal T-cell disorder of CD30+ cells. In contrast, Gellrich and coworkers[40]

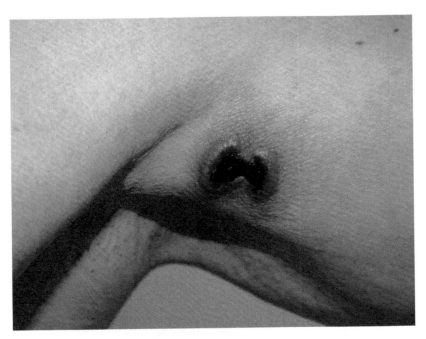

Fig. 7. LyP, type E: Angioinvasive growth of tumor cells resulting in eschar-like ulcer on the arm.

showed the polyclonal nature of CD30+ large atypical cells and assumed that those cells may not represent a uniform tumor cell population.

Chromosomal aberrations found in pcALCL and sALCL, such as t(2;5) (anaplastic lymphoma kinase–nucleophosmin [ALK-NPM]) or MUM1/IRF4 translocations are absent or present in only a small minority of LyP cases. Wada and colleagues[41] found IRF4 translocations in only 1 of 32 LyP cases (3%). The presence of the MUM1/IRF4 translocation does not correlate with the MUM1 expression detected by immunohistochemistry.[42] Recently, Karai and coworkers[43] identified a rare form of LyP with chromosomal rearrangements involving the DUSP22-IRF4 locus on 6p25.3. This variant manifested with localized lesions and histologically with prominent epidermotropism resembling pagetoid reticulosis overlying dense dermal infiltrates of small to medium-sized CD30+ lymphocytes.

DIFFERENTIAL DIAGNOSIS

The differential diagnosis of LyP is broad for 2 main reasons: (1) the wide spectrum of histologic manifestations of LyP, and (2) CD30 expression can be observed in a variety of CLs as well as systemic T-cell or B-cell lymphomas, but also in numerous reactive processes. Each histologic LyP type can mimic distinct CTCLs and even aggressive systemic lymphomas, as outlined in **Table 1**.

Distinction of cutaneous involvement by Hodgkin Lymphoma (HL) from LyP type A is based on the identification of underlying nodal HL via staging. CD15, a characteristic marker for Reed-Sternberg cells in HL, is expressed by atypical lymphocytes in half of LyP cases and is therefore not a useful marker for differential diagnosis.[44] The clinical presentation of MF with patches and plaques allow differentiation from LyP type B, which presents with papules and small nodules. Very rarely, MF presents with papular lesions. In those cases, papular lesions do not spontaneously regress as in LyP.

The histologic features of LyP type C and pcALCL, as well as sALCL are identical. To separate these entities, integration of clinical presentation, staging results, and phenotypic and genetic findings are mandatory. A comparison of features of LyP, pcALCL, and sALCL was presented by Diamantidis and Myrou.[45] Particularly CD8+ or CD56+ variants of LyP are prone to be misinterpreted as aggressive lymphomas. LyP type D needs to be distinguished from primary cutaneous CD8+ aggressive epidermotropic T-cell lymphoma (CD8+ AECTCL), which shows widespread erosive plaques and ulcerated nodules in contrast to the self-regressing papular lesions in LyP. Moreover, tumor cells in CD8+AECTCL express CD45RA and are consistently negative for CD30, whereas in LyP type D, CD30 is expressed by epidermotropic lymphocytes in 90% of the cases.[24] The angioinvasive growth pattern in LyP type E shares histologic features with cutaneous involvement by the angiocentric and angiodestructive variant of ALK-negative ALCL,[46] extranodal natural killer (NK)/T-cell lymphoma, nasal type, angiocentric cutaneous T-cell lymphoma of childhood (hydroa vacciniforme-like lymphoma), and cutaneous gamma/delta T-cell lymphoma (CGD-TCL), all of which can display CD30 expression.[47] The association with Epstein-Barr virus (EBV) and frequent systemic involvement in extranodal NK/T-cell lymphoma and hydroa vacciniforme-like lymphoma, and the immunohistochemical demonstration of TCR gamma expression in CGD-TCL are helpful in diagnosing these aggressive lymphomas and to differentiate them from LyP type E.[25,28]

Apart from CD30+ lymphomas, the number of inflammatory and infectious disorders that contain a significant number of CD30+ and sometimes atypical lymphocytes is steadily increasing and thereby expands the spectrum of simulators of CD30+ LPD.[8,48,49] CD30+ large cells are occasionally found in parapox virus infections, infestation-related infiltrates, and arthropod bite reactions.[8,9,48] Recent reports focused on drug reactions containing a significant number of CD30+ cells, thereby mimicking LyP type A. A broad variety of drugs can induce CD30+ drug eruptions, including carbamazepine, valsartan, or bortezomib (Fig. 8).[50] Varying combinations of spongiotic dermatitis, lichenoid infiltrates, and interface dermatitis were described with large atypical CD30+ lymphocytes accounting for 5% to 30% of all lymphocytes.[51] Lymphoma-associated and leukemia-associated cutaneous atypical CD30+ T-cell reactions represent eruptions after chemotherapy in patients with B-cell lymphoma and myeloid leukemia.[52] The perivascular infiltrates with highly atypical CD30+ lymphoid cells mimic recurrent lymphoma, but spontaneously resolve.

The lymphocytic infiltrate in pityriasis lichenoides et varioliformis acuta (PLEVA), a T-cell–mediated interface dermatitis of unknown etiology, can harbor a high number of CD30+ and either CD4+ or CD8+ T cells, thereby mimicking LyP type B or D (Fig. 9). Recently, we characterized the clinicopathological features of 13 patients with PLEVA harboring numerous CD30+ lymphocytes. In this series, more than half showed co-expression of CD8 and CD30 in the intraepidermal and dermal component of the infiltrate.[53] Moreover, monoclonal T cells were identified in 6 (55%) of 11 cases. In contrast to LyP, however, the lymphocytes in PLEVA did not exhibit significant atypia. Parakeratosis with exocytosis of small lymphocytes and vacuolization in the junctional zone are characteristic features of PLEVA, but vacuolization is not uncommon in LyP.[31] In our experience, clinico-pathologic correlation allows separation of CD30+ PLEVA from LyP in most, but not all cases. The overlap in histologic and phenotypic, as well as genotypic features in PLEVA and LyP suggest that these 2 disorders may be more closely related than traditional concepts suggest.[53,54]

In summary, diagnosis of LyP is based on the characteristic clinical presentation with waxing and waning of self-healing papulo-nodular lesions and the histologic and phenotypic findings. Self-healing is defined as spontaneous regression of each individual tumor lesion within weeks or months, whether or not new lesions occur. The histologic criteria of the 5 LyP types are summarized in Table 1. Among the various histologic types, LyP type B is particularly challenging to identify as a manifestation of LyP and thus may be underdiagnosed, as expression of CD30 is variable (and in some cases even absent) and its histology is indistinguishable from MF patch/plaque stage. Consequently, detailed clinical data are necessary to establish the diagnosis of LyP and to distinguish LyP type B from MF. In general, the overlapping histologic features of LyP with other CLs and even aggressive systemic lymphomas underline the necessity of clinicopathologic correlation as a crucial element in the diagnostic workup of CD30+ lymphoid infiltrates. Nevertheless, there is a small subset of patients in which LyP and pcALCL cannot be distinguished even by a careful clinicopathologic correlation. For those cases, the term borderline lesion is applied as outlined later in this article. This term also may be used to refer to a rapidly growing nodule that has a diameter larger than 1 cm in a patient with known LyP. Initially, it may be impossible to determine whether such a nodule merely reflects a larger lesion of LyP with the potential for spontaneous regression or the initial stage of pcALCL complicating LyP. In that situation, a tumor size of more than 2 cm and lack of spontaneous regression would indicate pcALCL.

According to recently published international recommendations for the management of CD30+ LPD, the recommended laboratory studies include a complete blood cell count with differential, blood chemistry, and lactate dehydrogenase (LDH).[7] In patients with the typical clinical manifestation of LyP, absence of enlarged lymph nodes, and negative blood tests, there is no need for radiologic staging examination or bone marrow biopsy. However, where physical examination or laboratory tests are suggestive of extracutaneous disease, radiologic examinations and lymph node biopsy (if enlarged lymph nodes are suspicious for nodal lymphoma) are recommended. It is still a matter of debate whether involvement of lymph nodes

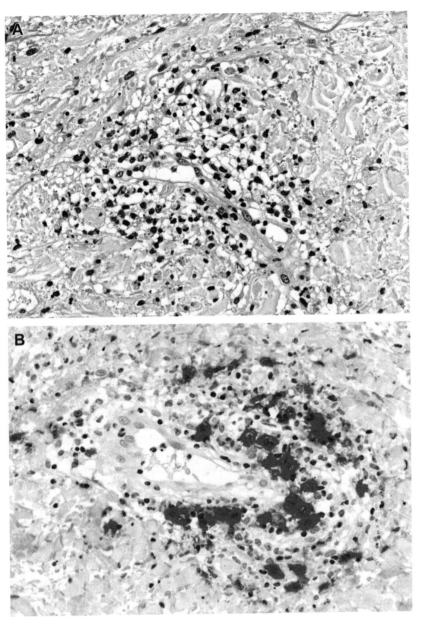

Fig. 8. CD30+ drug eruption: Lymphocytic vasculitis of small dermal vessels with lymphocytic nuclear dust (HE, original magnification ×100) (*A*) and medium-sized atypical CD30+ lymphocytes (*B*) (APAAP, original magnification ×200).

and viscera in LyP exists at all or whether occurrence of CD30+ lymphoma in lymph nodes and viscera should be regarded as concurrent nodal ALCL, even if clonally related to LyP. Considering the prognostic and therapeutic implications, it is important to differentiate secondary cutaneous involvement of sALCL from LyP by staging examinations and to identify underlying immunosuppressive conditions, as cutaneous CD30+ LPD arising in immunodeficient patients carry a worse

prognosis and may be treated with multiagent chemotherapy.

PROGNOSIS

LyP usually persists for years or even decades, but is not associated with mortality.[6,55] A subset of patients with LyP, however, develop a second lymphoid neoplasm, in particular MF, HL, and systemic or cutaneous ALCL. These lymphomas are

Fig. 9. Pityriasis lichenoides et varioliformis acuta (PLEVA): Exocytosis of numerous small lymphocytes, vacuolization in the junctional zone, apoptotic keratinocytes, and parakeratosis (*A*) (HE, original magnification ×100). Expression of CD30 by a subset of intraepidermal and dermal lymphocytes (*B*) (APAAP, original magnification ×200).

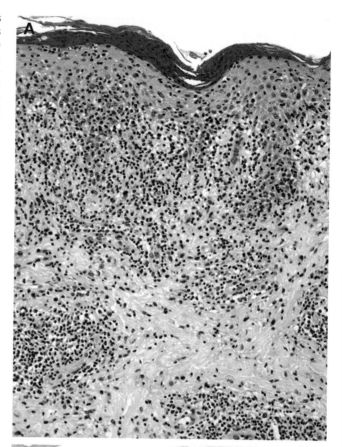

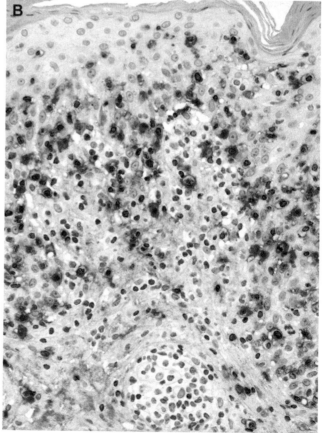

referred to as "LyP-associated malignant lymphomas" and can occur before, concurrent with, or after the manifestation of LyP. The prevalence of LyP-associated lymphomas reported in the literature widely varies, with a range of none to 62% of patients with LyP being affected (Table 2).[6,56–61] These divergent prevalence data may be due to geographic differences, differences in the age of the examined cohorts, or even result from an overrepresentation of patients with combinations of lymphoproliferative disorders. A clonal relationship between LyP and the associated lymphomas has been documented for some cases, which may indicate a common precursor for both neoplasms or a genetic defect in stem cells as underlying pathogenic factor.[62] Because of the lymphoma risk, patients with LyP should thus be monitored lifelong so that these potentially fatal lymphomas can be detected and treated early.

Remarkably, there are limited data on prognostic factors in LyP. We examined the expression of fascin, which is an actin-bundling protein expressed in HL, in biopsy specimens of patients with LyP with and without second lymphoid neoplasms and found that the expression of fascin by CD30+ large cells in LyP was significantly more common in cases with associated lymphomas (6/10 cases; 60%) than in uncomplicated LyP (11/45 cases; 24%).[63] Although expression of fascin could represent a prognostic factor, these data must be confirmed by additional studies. However, lack of fascin expression in individual cases of LyP does not exclude the risk for an associated lymphoma. Apart from fascin as a prognostic marker, monoclonal TCR gene rearrangement in LyP was reported in one study to be a prognostic indicator for the development of LyP-associated lymphomas.[31] Further studies on

risk factors for progression in LyP are urgently needed.

Because of its excellent prognosis, a "wait-and-see" strategy can be justified in the management of LyP, especially because so far no active therapeutic intervention has been proven to alter the course of the disease or to prevent LyP-associated lymphomas.[6,55] Multiagent chemotherapy should be avoided in LyP, because it is followed by rapid relapse of the disease in the vast majority of patients. For disseminated, numerous, or stigmatizing lesions, UV light–based therapy or low-dose methotrexate are the first-line therapies.[7]

PRIMARY CUTANEOUS ANAPLASTIC LARGE-CELL LYMPHOMA

OVERVIEW

ALCL refers to a T-cell lymphoma characterized by large lymphoid cells with prominent nuclear pleomorphism and expression of CD30 by more than 75% of tumor cells.[1,2,10] pcALCL was delineated as a distinct form of ALCL, as the course of pcALCL significantly differs from sALCL.[64] In addition, phenotypic and genetic studies showed major differences between pcALCL and sALCL.[5,65] Like LyP, pcALCL represents a paradox, because the favorable prognosis contrasts with the highly atypical cytomorphology of the CD30+ tumor cells and the rapid tumor growth. Recent studies have focused on new histologic and phenotypic variants, genetic characterization, and prognostic factors in pcALCL. Still unresolved issues are the lack of specific histologic or phenotypic markers to reliably distinguish pcALCL from the systemic form. Concerning treatment, surgical excision and radiotherapy represent well-documented first-line

Table 2
LyP-associated lymphomas: spectrum and frequency of second lymphomas in patients with lymphomatoid papulosis

Reference	LyP-associated Lymphomas	Hodgkin Lymphoma	Mycosis Fungoides	Anaplastic Large-Cell Lymphoma (Cutaneous or Systemic)
Thomsen & Wantzin,[56] 1987	7/30 (23%)	0	7	0
Wang et al,[57] 1992	16/57 (28%)	3	10	3 (NHL, NOS)
Christensen et al,[58] 1994	6/41 (15%)	1	3 (CTCL, NOS)	2
Bekkenk et al,[6] 2000	23/118 (19%)	2	11	10
Kunishige et al,[59] 2009	34/84 (40%)	2	16	15
Boccara et al,[60] 2012	0/24	0	0	0
Gan et al,[61] 2012	8/13 (62%)	0	7	1

Abbreviations: CTCL, cutaneous T-cell lymphoma; NHL, non-Hodgkin lymphoma; NOS, not otherwise specified.

therapies, but the best therapeutic strategy for multifocal pcALCL remains to be identified.

CLINICAL FEATURES

pcALCL presents with a solitary tumor or grouped firm nodules exhibiting rapid tumor growth. The tumors may reach a size of several centimeters and often show ulceration (**Fig. 10**). The head and neck and the extremities are predilection sites.[5] pcALCL mainly affects people in their sixth decade with a male-to-female ratio of 2 to 3:1, but it also can occur in childhood.[5,6,65] pcALCL is a common form of cutaneous T-cell lymphoma in HIV-infected individuals and organ transplant recipients.[66,67] Approximately 20% of the patients have multifocal disease with 2 or more lesions at different anatomic sites.[6,55] The tumors develop on normal skin without preceding patches or plaques, unlike MF in its tumor stage. Remarkably, spontaneous tumor regression is reported to occur in 10% to 42% of tumoral lesions in pcALCL.[6,7] In our experience, recurrences after spontaneous regression are common, and complete remission without therapeutic intervention is the exception.

DIAGNOSIS: MICROSCOPIC FEATURES

The archetypical histologic features in pcALCL are cohesive nodular infiltrates of large lymphoid cells extending into the deep dermis or subcutis. The large cells show a pleomorphic, anaplastic, or immunoblastic morphology with round, irregularly shaped nuclei, 1 or more nucleoli, and an abundant pale cytoplasm (**Fig. 11A, B**). Only a few neutrophils or eosinophils are present. Epidermotropism is usually absent or subtle. Ulceration may be present.

Neutrophil-rich and eosinophil-rich forms of the disease are more commonly found in immunodeficient patients and may pose a diagnostic problem, because the tumor cells may be obscured by numerous neutrophils or eosinophils.[68] Release of interleukin (IL)-8, a potent chemoattractant for neutrophils, by tumor cells best explains the neutrophil-rich infiltrates. IL-8 was found at exceedingly high levels in patients' sera and in the supernatant of cultured tumor cells in vitro.[69] The neutrophil-rich variant of pcALCL may clinically and histologically be misinterpreted as pyoderma gangrenosum. The pseudoepitheliomatous epidermal hyperplasia overlying the infiltrates of CD30+ tumor cells is the hallmark of the keratoacanthoma-like variant of pcALCL.[70,71] Other unusual presentations are an angiocentric and/or angiodestructive growth pattern, and subcutaneous ALCL (**Fig. 12**).[72,73] In addition, a small-cell variant of ALCL has been identified.[74] In a study by Massone and colleagues,[72] cases composed predominantly of small to medium-sized CD30+ tumor cells accounted for one-quarter of all biopsies. The sarcomatoid variant of pcALCL is very rare and shows a prominent spindle-cell

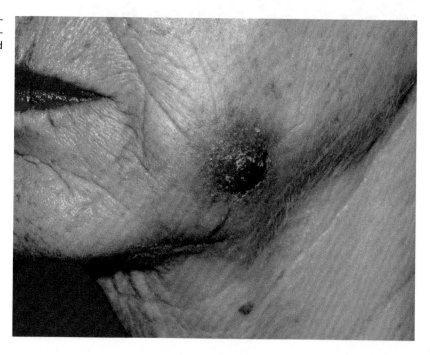

Fig. 10. Primary cutaneous anaplastic large-cell lymphoma: Ulcerated nodule on the face.

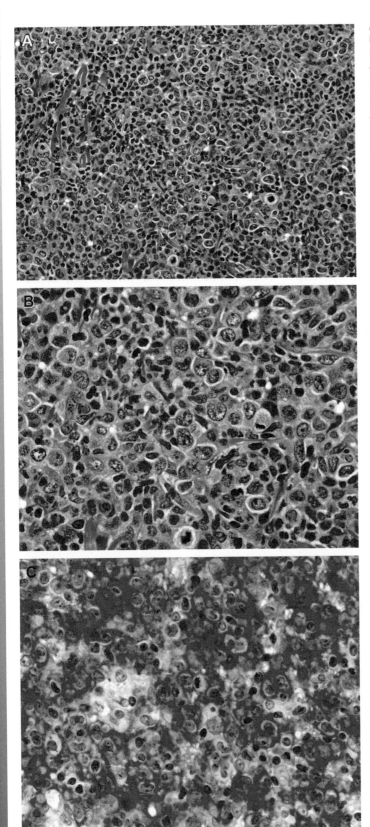

Fig. 11. Primary cutaneous anaplastic large-cell lymphoma: Dense cohesive infiltrates of large pleomorphic and anaplastic lymphoid cells (A: HE, original magnification ×200; B: HE, original magnification ×400) (A, B). There is prominent nuclear pleomorphism of tumor cells (B) and CD30 expression (C) (APAAP, original magnification ×400).

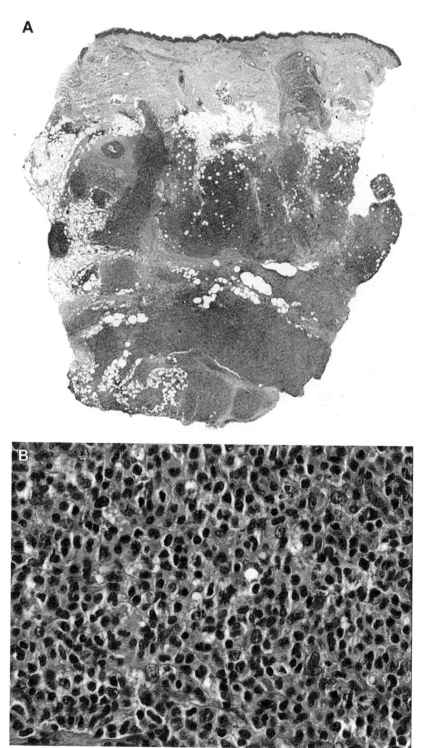

Fig. 12. Subcutaneous variant of anaplastic large-cell lymphoma: Dense, mostly lobular pannicular lymphocytic infiltrates (HE, original magnification ×10) (*A*) of medium-sized to large CD30+ tumor cells (HE, original magnification ×400) (*B*). (*Courtesy of* Dr U. Hillen, Essen, Germany.)

morphology, thereby mimicking spindle-cell sarcomas.[75] An unusual form of ALCL that may involve the skin is the intravascular variant of ALCL (IV-ALCL). Clinically, IV-ALCL manifests with patches and plaques or nodular lesions.[76,77] In contrast to the other T-cell variants of intravascular lymphoma, the anaplastic tumor cells express CD4 and CD30, but are negative for cytotoxic markers and Epstein-Barr virus encoded small RNA (EBER). ALK-1 and epithelial membrane antigen (EMA) are rarely expressed in IV-ALCL. The data on prognosis of IV-ALCL are heterogeneous and do not allow one to draw stringent conclusions.

In all histologic forms of pcALCL, the tumor cells are highlighted and identifiable by the expression of CD30, which demonstrates the importance of immunohistochemistry in the diagnosis of pcALCL.

DIAGNOSIS: ANCILLARY STUDIES

The hallmark of pcALCL is the expression of CD30 by at least 75% of the tumor cells as defined in the current WHO classification (**Fig. 11C**).[10] The tumor cells in pcALCL carry an activated T-cell phenotype with expression of T-cell–associated antigens CD2, CD4, and CD45RO and variable loss of T-cell antigens (CD2 and CD5).[5,65] CD3 may be absent or expressed at a lower level than in other cutaneous T-cell lymphomas and reactive small T-cells due to genetic alterations in the TCR coding regions on chromosome 1.[78] In addition to CD30, the tumor cells exhibit other activation markers, such as CD25 (IL-2R), CD71, and HLA-DR, and at least one cytotoxic protein (such as TIA-1, granzyme B, and perforin) is expressed in about half of pcALCLs.[79] Different from sALCL, pcALCL shows only focally or lacks expression of EMA, but exhibits the cutaneous lymphocyte antigen (CLA, HECA-452). Along with ALK and EMA, other markers, such as HOXC5, appear to be differentially expressed in nodal and cutaneous ALCL, but the latter is not widely available for diagnosis.[80] There are T-cell and null-cell variants of ALCL. Rare B-cell forms have been described in HIV-infected patients but are now considered to be anaplastic variants of diffuse large B-cell lymphoma.[64]

In pcALCL, clonal rearrangement of TCR genes can be found in 90% of the cases.[81] In neutrophil-rich and eosinophil-rich forms of pcALCL, however, clonality assays may fail to detect a clonal tumor cell population, possibly due to the under-representation of tumor-cell DNA, even when using very sensitive PCR-based methods.[68,69]

The genetic signature of pcALCL demonstrates that pcALCL is distinct from other forms of ALCL. The translocation t(2;5)(p23;q35) involving ALK-NPM genes is found in about 60% of sALCLs, but is present in only a rare subset (less than 10%) of pcALCLs.[82] Thus, its presence in cutaneous CD30+ large-cell infiltrates should raise suspicion for secondary cutaneous involvement by sALCL. Recently, rare and unusual cases of ALK-positive pcALCL were described and were associated with a variant translocation and cytoplasmic staining of ALK.[83,84] The course of ALK-positive pcALCL has been heterogeneous, with some cases showing a more aggressive course. On the other hand, Oschlies and coworkers[85] described a series of 6 children with ALK-positive ALCL limited to the skin with complete remission and excellent prognosis. Further studies are needed to clarify the biology of this peculiar variant of pcALCL. From a therapeutic point of view, the identification of ALK expression or the underlying translocation is important because those patients could benefit from the treatment with the ALK inhibitor crizotinib.[86]

pcALCL may share histologic features with peripheral T-cell lymphoma, not otherwise specified (PTL-NOS), but differs with regard to CD30 expression and genetic alterations (for review see Ref.[87]). Although both pcALCL and PTL-NOS harbor gains on chromosome 7q and 17q, pcALCL displays gains on chromosome 7q and 17q and losses on 6q and 13q. It thereby differs from PTL-NOS carrying gains on chromosome 8 and loss on 9p21.[88] Rearrangements of the IRF4-DUSP22 locus on 6p25.3 were identified in 28% of pcALCLs.[41,89] Interestingly, detection of 6p25.3 rearrangement by fluorescence in situ hybridization is a highly specific marker for pcALCL, with a specificity of 99%.[41]

The higher expression of the skin-homing chemokine receptor genes CCR10 and CCR8 in pcALCL may explain the lower tendency to disseminate to extracutaneous sites compared with the aggressive PTL-NOS.[88] Regarding the expression of micro RNA (miRNA), recent data indicate an expression pattern in pcALCL different from tumor stage MF.[90]

DIFFERENTIAL DIAGNOSIS

The differential diagnosis of pcALCL includes a broad range of primary cutaneous and systemic lymphoproliferations with large-cell morphology and expression of CD30 by most tumor cells. As outlined previously, there is no histologic or phenotypic marker allowing distinction between LyP type C and pcALCL; these entities differ with regard to the clinical presentation and the life cycle of the lesions. Recently, the expression of chemokine receptors has been investigated; expression of CXCR3 was found in most LyP cases, but in none of the 4 ALCL cases.[91] However, these data must be confirmed by further studies before the expression pattern of chemokine receptors can be used for diagnostic purposes. The large tumor cells in transformed MF commonly express CD30 at a variable degree, but only a subset shows expression of CD30 by more than half of the large cells. Those cases can perfectly mimic ALCL; however, the clinical presentation of MF with patches and plaques preceding tumor stage readily allows separating MF from pcALCL. Analogous to MF, transformation to large-cell lymphoma also can occur in Sézary syndrome, either in the skin or in the lymph nodes, and therefore must be included in the list of differential diagnoses.[92] Cutaneous PTL-NOS may share cytomorphological features and nodular growth pattern with pcALCL, but CD30 is absent or expressed by only a minority of the tumor cells.[87] To differentiate PTL-NOS from pcALCL is essential considering the unfavorable prognosis of PTL-NOS and the therapeutic implications. Future studies will help clarify whether the differences in the miRNA pattern between pcALCL and transformed MF and the genetic differences between pcALCL and PTL-NOS mentioned above can be used for diagnostic purposes.[88,90]

Among systemic lymphomas, distinction from sALCL is very important considering the prognostic and therapeutic impact. The expression of ALK, which is found in 60% of sALCLs, should raise suspicion for secondary cutaneous involvement. On the other hand, expression of cutaneous lymphocyte-associated antigen (CLA) is typically present in pcALCL, but not in sALCL. Adult T-cell lymphoma/leukemia (ATLL) may be included in the differential diagnosis, as this lymphoma can present with cohesive infiltrates of medium to large pleomorphic cells and expression of CD30. Detection of HTLV-1 sequences integrated into the tumor cell genome and clinicopathologic features are crucial to distinguish the so-called lymphomatous stage of ATLL from pcALCL. Angiocentric and angiodestructive ALCL differs from CD30+ extranodal NK/T-cell lymphoma, nasal type by the lack of EBV.[47] In addition, staging is mandatory to separate pcALCL from the previously listed systemic lymphomas.

Furthermore, one should keep in mind that expression of CD30 is not restricted to lymphocytic neoplasms, but also may occur in histiocytic disorders, such as reticulohistiocytoma, Langerhans cell histiocytosis, and systemic mastocytosis, as well as in benign reactive processes. Benign atypical intravascular CD30+ T-cell proliferation represents a recently described reactive condition.[93,94] It shows an accumulation of CD30 large lymphocytes in the lymphatics beneath ulcers in chronically inflamed skin (Fig. 13) and may mimic intravascular T-cell or NK/T-cell lymphoma and the rare intravascular form of sALCL.[95] In contrast to intravascular ALCL, the intravascular CD30+ lymphocytes have nuclei with dense chromatin and lack mitotic activity.

The clinical and histologic criteria of pcALCL are listed in Box 1. The distinction of pcALCL from LyP and CD30+ large cell transformation of MF is based on clinical grounds. Some features would raise suspicion of secondary cutaneous involvement by sALCL, such as multifocal lesions, small-cell and neutrophil-rich or eosinophil-rich forms, and expression of ALK. Especially in neutrophil-rich and eosinophil-rich forms, underlying immunodeficiency, in particular HIV infection, should be excluded. Staging is essential to separate pcALCL from secondary cutaneous involvement by sALCL, especially because no single histologic, phenotypic, or genetic marker allows one to reliably distinguish pcALCL from sALCL, as discussed previously. With regard to radiologic staging, positron emission tomography in combination with computerized tomography (PET-CT) is becoming more widely used and has largely replaced conventional CT in the radiologic workup. A retrospective analysis on a large series of patients with pcALCL indicated that bone marrow biopsy is of limited value.[96] Based on these data, bone marrow biopsy is no longer considered to be mandatory, especially in patients with negative radiologic staging.[7,96]

PROGNOSIS

In contrast to systemic lymphomas, pcALCL has a favorable prognosis with a 5-year survival rate between 76% and 96%.[6,97] pcALCL arising on the legs showed an impaired prognosis, with a 5-year survival rate of 76%.[97] Extensive limb involvement and progression to extracutaneous disease are independent prognostic factors for disease-specific survival.[98] Presentation with T3 disease was identified as a risk factor for progression to extracutaneous disease. Remarkably, microarray analysis revealed in that study that patients with pcALCL with extensive limb involvement had a differential gene expression profile and formed distinct clusters.[98] Involvement of locoregional lymph nodes seems not to be associated with a worse prognosis than cutaneous involvement alone, but these data are based on only one study of a limited number of patients and need to be confirmed in future studies.[6] Skin-limited relapses of pcALCL were observed in 39% of

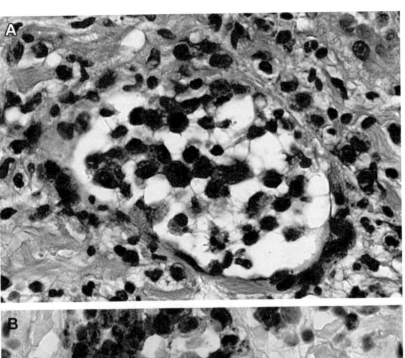

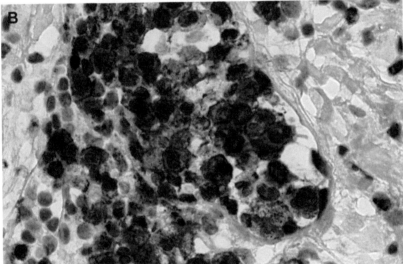

Fig. 13. Benign intravascular atypical CD30+ T-cell proliferation: Intralymphatic accumulation of atypical lymphocytes (HE, original magnification ×400) (*A*) with expression of CD30 (*B*) (APAAP, original magnification ×400).

patients, and extracutaneous spread in 13% of the patients.[99] In contrast to immunocompetent individuals, immunosuppressed patients with pcALCL are confronted with a more aggressive course of the disease and a worse prognosis.[100,101]

Surgical excision and radiotherapy are recommended first-line therapies for solitary or grouped pcALCL.[7] Multiagent chemotherapy is indicated only for extracutaneous tumor spread beyond locoregional lymph nodes. The best treatment for multifocal pcALCL has not yet been determined,

as there is only anecdotal data for the previously reported therapeutic approaches.

BORDERLINE LESIONS

The term "borderline lesions" was introduced to designate cases in which, despite careful clinicopathologic correlation, a definite distinction between LyP and pcALCL cannot be made at the time of diagnosis.[1,7] It can be challenging and in some cases even impossible to differentiate between LyP and pcALCL in patients presenting

> **Box 1**
> **Primary cutaneous anaplastic large cell lymphoma: diagnostic criteria**
>
> Clinical criteria:
>
> - Solitary, grouped, or multifocal nodular lesions
>
> - No clinical evidence of lymphomatoid papulosis, mycosis fungoides, or other types of cutaneous T-cell lymphomas.
>
> Histologic criteria:
>
> - Dense nodular dermal infiltrate composed of large pleomorphic, anaplastic, or immunoblastic cells with large, irregularly shaped nuclei and abundant pale or eosinophilic cytoplasm.
>
> - Clusters of small reactive lymphocytes and eosinophils may be found within and surrounding the tumor cells.
>
> Immunophenotypical criteria:
>
> - Expression of CD30 by at least 75% of tumor cells.
>
> - Expression of CD4 or CD8 in most cases with variable loss of pan-T-cell antigens (CD2, CD3, CD5).
>
> - ALK-1 (p80) and t(2;5) translocation are usually absent.
>
> Staging procedures:
>
> No evidence of extracutaneous lymphoma manifestation.
>
> *Adapted from* Kempf W, Pfaltz K, Vermeer MH, et al. EORTC, ISCL, and USCLC consensus recommendations for the treatment of primary cutaneous CD30-positive lymphoproliferative disorders: lymphomatoid papulosis and primary cutaneous anaplastic large-cell lymphoma. Blood 2011;118(15):4024–35.

with a short history of multifocal papulo-nodular lesions. Moreover, spontaneous regression of individual tumors is a hallmark of LyP, but also has been observed in patients with multifocal pcALCL as well. The term borderline lesion, however, is generally regarded as a working diagnosis. In most cases, the final diagnosis can be achieved during follow-up based on clinical behavior.

CD30 AS PROGNOSTIC MARKER AND EXPRESSION IN OTHER LYMPHOMAS

As outlined previously, the expression of CD30 by tumor cells is not limited to the group of cutaneous CD30+ LPDs and sALCLs. Whereas in cutaneous CD30+ LPD, the expression of CD30 indicates a favorable prognosis, CD30 has a divergent prognostic impact in other lymphomas. In patch and plaque-stage MF, the presence of CD30+ dermal lymphocytes and a high proliferation rate have been linked to impaired prognosis.[12] This scenario has to be distinguished from transformed MF, which refers to the occurrence of large tumor cells accounting for more than 25% of the entire lymphocytic infiltrate. In transformed MF, expression of CD30 by large cells is associated with a longer survival than in CD30– cases.[102] So far, no conclusive data have been reported on the impact of CD30 expression in other forms of CL. The prognostic differences in various disease stages of

MF depending on CD30 and the lack of conclusive data on the prognostic impact of CD30 in other lymphomas make the prognostic significance of CD30 expression a rather complex issue.

Although expression of CD30 by tumor cells is most commonly observed in T-cell non-Hodgkin lymphomas (NHLs), it also has been observed in cutaneous and systemic B-cell lymphomas. Scattered CD30+ blasts are regularly found in primary cutaneous marginal zone lymphoma.[103] The expression of CD30 by tumor cells in low-grade indolent forms of cutaneous B-cell lymphomas, however, is a very rare event. Based on the data in the literature and our own experience on 4 cases of CD30+ primary cutaneous follicle center lymphoma (pcFCL), CD30 has no prognostic impact in pcFCL and is not linked to EBV.[104] In B-cell NHL composed of large tumor cells, such as diffuse large B-cell lymphoma, plasmablastic lymphoma, or posttransplant lymphoproliferative disorders, expression of CD30 often goes along with EBV infection and underlying immunodeficiency.[105,106] These forms of B-NHL are aggressive and should not be misinterpreted as indolent lymphomas based on the CD30 expression by tumor cells.

CD30 AS THERAPEUTIC MARKER

CD30 is an ideal antigen for targeted therapy because of its preferential expression on tumor cells and only occasional presence on other cells under physiologic conditions. Binding of CD30L to its receptor on CD30+ tumor cells exerts divergent actions in different forms of CD30+ T-cell lymphomas resulting either in apoptosis or proliferation of cultured tumor cells. Nevertheless, treatment with anti-CD30 antibody alone has shown efficacy in sALCL and HL, but also in small series of cutaneous CD30+ LPDs.[107] Recently, anti-CD30 antibodies conjugated to cytotoxic agents, such as brentuximab vedotin, have been approved for sALCL and HL and are currently being studied in cutaneous CD30+ LPD, as well as in other types of CTCL with variable expression of CD30.[108] Interestingly, response to the drug does not correlate with the presence and level of CD30 expression assessed by immunohistochemistry, as MF cases with only a few CD30+ cells also have responded to this therapeutic strategy.[11] In those cases with only a few CD30+ cells, other pathways could be implied and mediate the efficacy of the anti-CD30 antibody. Nevertheless, standardized immunohistochemical staining protocols may be needed, especially because quality-control studies, such as the Nordic Immunohistochemical Quality Control (NordiQC) study, have revealed variations in the detection and expression levels among different laboratories (for review see Ref.[109]). Criteria for optimal staining have been proposed and underscore the necessity of appropriate positive controls when performing immunohistochemistry (IHC) for CD30.[109] In addition, these observations raise the question of whether IHC alone is sufficient to properly assess CD30 expression in the tumor tissue or whether analysis should be performed by flow cytometry or molecular assays, such as in situ hybridization or quantitative PCR, for CD30 mRNA. In the future, standardized immunohistochemical protocols and an improved molecular profiling of CD30+ LPD are needed for diagnostic purposes and to assess the prognosis of these lymphomas in individual patients.

REFERENCES

1. Willemze R, Jaffe ES, Burg G, et al. WHO-EORTC classification for cutaneous lymphomas. Blood 2005;105(10):3768–85.
2. Kempf W, Willemze R, Jaffe ES, et al. CD30+ T-cell lymphoproliferative disorders. In: LeBoit P, Burg G, Weedon D, et al, editors. World Health Organization classification of tumours. Pathology and genetics of skin tumours. Lyon (France): IARC Press; 2006. p. 179–81.
3. Stein H, Mason DY, Gerdes J, et al. The expression of the Hodgkin's disease associated antigen Ki-1 in reactive and neoplastic lymphoid tissue: evidence that Reed-Sternberg cells and histiocytic malignancies are derived from activated lymphoid cells. Blood 1985;66(4):848–58.
4. Kadin ME, Levi E, Kempf W. Progression of lymphomatoid papulosis to systemic lymphoma is associated with escape from growth inhibition by transforming growth factor-beta and CD30 ligand. Ann N Y Acad Sci 2001;941:59–68.
5. Kadin ME, Carpenter C. Systemic and primary cutaneous anaplastic large cell lymphomas. Semin Hematol 2003;40(3):244–56.
6. Bekkenk MW, Geelen FA, van Voorst Vader PC, et al. Primary and secondary cutaneous CD30(+) lymphoproliferative disorders: a report from the Dutch Cutaneous Lymphoma Group on the long-term follow-up data of 219 patients and guidelines for diagnosis and treatment. Blood 2000;95(12):3653–61.
7. Kempf W, Pfaltz K, Vermeer MH, et al. EORTC, ISCL, and USCLC consensus recommendations for the treatment of primary cutaneous CD30-positive lymphoproliferative disorders: lymphomatoid papulosis and primary cutaneous anaplastic large-cell lymphoma. Blood 2011;118(15):4024–35.
8. Kempf W. CD30+ lymphoproliferative disorders: histopathology, differential diagnosis, new variants, and simulators. J Cutan Pathol 2006;33(Suppl 1):58–70.
9. Werner B, Massone C, Kerl H, et al. Large CD30-positive cells in benign, atypical lymphoid infiltrates of the skin. J Cutan Pathol 2008;35(12):1100–7.
10. Swerdlow SH, Campo E, Harris NL, et al. WHO classification of tumours of haematopoietic and lymphoid tissues. 4th edition. Lyon (France): IARC Press; 2008.
11. Duvic M. CD30+ neoplasms of the skin. Curr Hematol Malig Rep 2011;6(4):245–50.
12. Edinger JT, Clark BZ, Pucevich BE, et al. CD30 expression and proliferative fraction in nontransformed mycosis fungoides. Am J Surg Pathol 2009;33(12):1860–8.
13. Macaulay WL. Lymphomatoid papulosis. A continuing self-healing eruption, clinically benign–histologically malignant. Arch Dermatol 1968;97(1):23–30.
14. Burgdorf W, Kempf W, Warren L. Macaulay (1915-2006)—in memoriam. J Am Acad Dermatol 2006;55:730–2.
15. Zirbel GM, Gellis SE, Kadin ME, et al. Lymphomatoid papulosis in children. J Am Acad Dermatol 1995;33(5 Pt 1):741–8.
16. Nijsten T, Curiel-Lewandrowski C, Kadin ME. Lymphomatoid papulosis in children: a retrospective cohort study of 35 cases. Arch Dermatol 2004;140(3):306–12.

17. Scarisbrick JJ, Evans AV, Woolford AJ, et al. Regional lymphomatoid papulosis: a report of four cases. Br J Dermatol 1999;141(6):1125–8.

18. Barnadas MA, Lopez D, Pujol RM, et al. Pustular lymphomatoid papulosis in childhood. J Am Acad Dermatol 1992;27(4):627–8.

19. Kempf W, Kazakov DV, Baumgartner HP, et al. Follicular lymphomatoid papulosis revisited: a study of 11 cases, with new histopathological findings. J Am Acad Dermatol 2013;68(5): 809–16.

20. Pileri A, Bacci F, Neri I, et al. Persistent agmination of lymphomatoid papulosis: an ongoing debate. Dermatology 2012;225(2):131–4.

21. Pujol RM, Muret MP, Bergua P, et al. Oral involvement in lymphomatoid papulosis. Report of two cases and review of the literature. Dermatology 2005;210(1):53–7.

22. Salisbury CL, Budnick SD, Li S. T-cell receptor gene rearrangement and CD30 immunoreactivity in traumatic ulcerative granuloma with stromal eosinophilia of the oral cavity. Am J Clin Pathol 2009;132(5):722–7.

23. El Shabrawi-Caelen L, Kerl H, Cerroni L. Lymphomatoid papulosis: reappraisal of clinicopathologic presentation and classification into subtypes A, B, and C. Arch Dermatol 2004;140(4):441–7.

24. Saggini A, Gulia A, Argenyi Z, et al. A variant of lymphomatoid papulosis simulating primary cutaneous aggressive epidermotropic CD8+ cytotoxic T-cell lymphoma. Description of 9 cases. Am J Surg Pathol 2010;34(8):1168–75.

25. Kempf W, Kazakov DV, Scharer L, et al. Angioinvasive lymphomatoid papulosis: a new variant simulating aggressive lymphomas. Am J Surg Pathol 2013;37(1):1–13.

26. Cardoso J, Duhra P, Thway Y, et al. Lymphomatoid papulosis type D: a newly described variant easily confused with cutaneous aggressive CD8-positive cytotoxic T-cell lymphoma. Am J Dermatopathol 2012;34(7):762–5.

27. Bertolotti A, Pham-Ledard AL, Vergier B, et al. Lymphomatoid papulosis type D: an aggressive histology for an indolent disease. Br J Dermatol 2013;169(5):1157–9.

28. Sharaf MA, Romanelli P, Kirsner R, et al. Angioinvasive lymphomatoid papulosis: another case of a newly described variant. Am J Dermatopathol 2014;36:e75–7.

29. Requena L, Sanchez M, Coca S, et al. Follicular lymphomatoid papulosis. Am J Dermatopathol 1990;12(1):67–75.

30. Crowson AN, Baschinsky DY, Kovatich A, et al. Granulomatous eccrinotropic lymphomatoid papulosis. Am J Clin Pathol 2003;119(5):731–9.

31. de Souza A, el-Azhary RA, Camilleri MJ, et al. In search of prognostic indicators for lymphomatoid papulosis: a retrospective study of 123 patients. J Am Acad Dermatol 2012;66(6):928–37.

32. Varga FJ, Vonderheid EC, Olbricht SM, et al. Immunohistochemical distinction of lymphomatoid papulosis and pityriasis lichenoides et varioliformis acuta. Am J Pathol 1990;136(4):979–87.

33. de Souza A, Camilleri MJ, Wada DA, et al. Clinical, histopathologic, and immunophenotypic features of lymphomatoid papulosis with CD8 predominance in 14 pediatric patients. J Am Acad Dermatol 2009;61(6):993–1000.

34. Bekkenk MW, Kluin PM, Jansen PM, et al. Lymphomatoid papulosis with a natural killer-cell phenotype. Br J Dermatol 2001;145(2):318–22.

35. Kummer JA, Vermeer MH, Dukers D, et al. Most primary cutaneous CD30-positive lymphoproliferative disorders have a CD4-positive cytotoxic T-cell phenotype. J Invest Dermatol 1997;109(5): 636–40.

36. Morimura S, Sugaya M, Tamaki Z, et al. Lymphomatoid papulosis showing gammadelta T-cell phenotype. Acta Derm Venereol 2011;91(6):712–3.

37. Rodriguez-Pinilla SM, Ortiz-Romero PL, Monsalvez V, et al. TCR-gamma expression in primary cutaneous T-cell lymphomas. Am J Surg Pathol 2013;37(3):375–84.

38. Greisser J, Palmedo G, Sander C, et al. Detection of clonal rearrangement of T-cell receptor genes in the diagnosis of primary cutaneous CD30 lymphoproliferative disorders. J Cutan Pathol 2006; 33(11):711–5.

39. Steinhoff M, Hummel M, Anagnostopoulos I, et al. Single-cell analysis of CD30+ cells in lymphomatoid papulosis demonstrates a common clonal T-cell origin. Blood 2002;100(2):578–84.

40. Gellrich S, Wernicke M, Wilks A, et al. The cell infiltrate in lymphomatoid papulosis comprises a mixture of polyclonal large atypical cells (CD30-positive) and smaller monoclonal T cells (CD30-negative). J Invest Dermatol 2004;122(3):859–61.

41. Wada DA, Law ME, Hsi ED, et al. Specificity of IRF4 translocations for primary cutaneous anaplastic large cell lymphoma: a multicenter study of 204 skin biopsies. Mod Pathol 2011;24(4):596–605.

42. Kiran T, Demirkesen C, Eker C, et al. The significance of MUM1/IRF4 protein expression and IRF4 translocation of CD30(+) cutaneous T-cell lymphoproliferative disorders: a study of 53 cases. Leuk Res 2013;37(4):396–400.

43. Karai LJ, Kadin ME, Hsi ED, et al. Chromosomal rearrangements of 6p25.3 define a new subtype of lymphomatoid papulosis. Am J Surg Pathol 2013; 37(8):1173–81.

44. Moreau Cabarrot A, Bonafe JL, Gorguet B, et al. Papulose lymphomatoide et lymphome anaplasique a grandes cellules. Ann Dermatol Venereol 1994;121(10):727–30.

45. Diamantidis MD, Myrou AD. Perils and pitfalls regarding differential diagnosis and treatment of primary cutaneous anaplastic large-cell lymphoma. ScientificWorldJournal 2011;11:1048–55.

46. Nambudiri VE, Aboutalebi A, Granter SR, et al. Recurrent ALK-negative anaplastic large T-cell lymphoma presenting as necrotizing vasculitis. Am J Dermatopathol 2013;35(4):512–6.

47. Ferenczi K, Summers P, Aubert P, et al. A case of CD30+ nasal natural killer/T-cell lymphoma. Am J Dermatopathol 2008;30(6):567–71.

48. Guitart J, Querfeld C. Cutaneous CD30 lymphoproliferative disorders and similar conditions: a clinical and pathologic prospective on a complex issue. Semin Diagn Pathol 2009;26(3):131–40.

49. Sarantopoulos GP, Palla B, Said J, et al. Mimics of cutaneous lymphoma: report of the 2011 Society for Hematopathology/European Association for Haematopathology workshop. Am J Clin Pathol 2013;139(4):536–51.

50. Garcia-Navarro X, Puig L, Fernandez-Figueras MT, et al. Bortezomib-associated cutaneous vasculitis. Br J Dermatol 2007;157(4):799–801.

51. Pulitzer MP, Nolan KA, Oshman RG, et al. CD30+ lymphomatoid drug reactions. Am J Dermatopathol 2013;35(3):343–50.

52. Su LD, Duncan LM. Lymphoma- and leukemia-associated cutaneous atypical CD30+ T-cell reactions. J Cutan Pathol 2000;27(5):249–54.

53. Kempf W, Kazakov DV, Palmedo G, et al. Pityriasis lichenoides et varioliformis acuta with numerous CD30+ cells: a variant mimicking lymphomatoid papulosis and other cutaneous lymphomas. A clinicopathologic, immunohistochemical, and molecular biological study of 13 cases. Am J Surg Pathol 2012;36(7):1021–9.

54. Vonderheid EC, Kadin ME, Gocke CD. Lymphomatoid papulosis followed by pityriasis lichenoides: a common pathogenesis? Am J Dermatopathol 2011;33(8):835–40.

55. Paulli M, Berti E, Rosso R, et al. CD30/Ki-1-positive lymphoproliferative disorders of the skin—clinicopathologic correlation and statistical analysis of 86 cases: a multicentric study from the European Organization for Research and Treatment of Cancer Cutaneous Lymphoma Project Group. J Clin Oncol 1995;13(6):1343–54.

56. Thomsen K, Wantzin GL. Lymphomatoid papulosis. A follow-up study of 30 patients. J Am Acad Dermatol 1987;17(4):632–6.

57. Wang HH, Lach L, Kadin ME. Epidemiology of lymphomatoid papulosis. Cancer 1992;70(12):2951–7.

58. Christensen HK, Thomsen K, Vejlsgaard GL. Lymphomatoid papulosis: a follow-up study of 41 patients. Semin Dermatol 1994;13(3):197–201.

59. Kunishige JH, McDonald H, Alvarez G, et al. Lymphomatoid papulosis and associated lymphomas: a retrospective case series of 84 patients. Clin Exp Dermatol 2009;34(5):576–81.

60. Boccara O, Blanche S, de Prost Y, et al. Cutaneous hematologic disorders in children. Pediatr Blood Cancer 2012;58(2):226–32.

61. Gan EY, Tang MB, Tan SH. Lymphomatoid papulosis: is a second lymphoma commoner among East Asians? Clin Exp Dermatol 2012;37(2):118–21.

62. Davis TH, Morton CC, Miller Cassman R, et al. Hodgkin's disease, lymphomatoid papulosis, and cutaneous T-cell lymphoma derived from a common T-cell clone. N Engl J Med 1992;326(17):1115–22.

63. Kempf W, Levi E, Kamarashev J, et al. Fascin expression in CD30-positive cutaneous lymphoproliferative disorders. J Cutan Pathol 2002;29(5):295–300.

64. Fornari A, Piva R, Chiarle R, et al. Anaplastic large cell lymphoma: one or more entities among T-cell lymphoma? Hematol Oncol 2009;27(4):161–70.

65. Stein H, Foss HD, Durkop H, et al. CD30(+) anaplastic large cell lymphoma: a review of its histopathologic, genetic, and clinical features. Blood 2000;96(12):3681–95.

66. Kerschmann RL, Berger TG, Weiss LM, et al. Cutaneous presentations of lymphoma in human immunodeficiency virus disease. Predominance of T cell lineage. Arch Dermatol 1995;131(11):1281–8.

67. Yurtsever H, Kempf W, Laeng RH. Posttransplant CD30+ anaplastic large cell lymphoma with skin and lymph node involvement. Dermatology 2003;207(1):107–10.

68. Mann KP, Hall B, Kamino H, et al. Neutrophil-rich, Ki-1-positive anaplastic large-cell malignant lymphoma. Am J Surg Pathol 1995;19(4):407–16.

69. Burg G, Kempf W, Kazakov DV, et al. Pyogenic lymphoma of the skin: a peculiar variant of primary cutaneous neutrophil-rich CD30+ anaplastic large-cell lymphoma. Clinicopathological study of four cases and review of the literature. Br J Dermatol 2003;148(3):580–6.

70. Lin JH, Lee JY. Primary cutaneous CD30 anaplastic large cell lymphoma with keratoacanthoma-like pseudocarcinomatous hyperplasia and marked eosinophilia and neutrophilia. J Cutan Pathol 2004;31(6):458–61.

71. Resnik KS, Kutzner H. Of lymphocytes and cutaneous epithelium: keratoacanthomatous hyperplasia in CD30+ lymphoproliferative disorders and CD30+ cells associated with keratoacanthoma. Am J Dermatopathol 2010;32(3):314–5.

72. Massone C, El-Shabrawi-Caelen L, Kerl H, et al. The morphologic spectrum of primary cutaneous anaplastic large T-cell lymphoma: a histopathologic study on 66 biopsy specimens from 47 patients with report of rare variants. J Cutan Pathol 2008;35(1):46–53.

73. Kempf W, Kazakov DV, Paredes BE, et al. Primary cutaneous anaplastic large cell lymphoma with angioinvasive features and cytotoxic phenotype: a rare lymphoma variant within the spectrum of CD30+ lymphoproliferative disorders. Dermatology 2013;227(4):346–52.

74. Kinney MC, Collins RD, Greer JP, et al. A small-cell-predominant variant of primary Ki-1 (CD30)+ T-cell lymphoma. Am J Surg Pathol 1993;17(9):859–68.

75. Wang J, Sun NC, Nozawa Y, et al. Histological and immunohistochemical characterization of extranodal diffuse large-cell lymphomas with prominent spindle cell features. Histopathology 2001;39(5): 476–81.

76. Iacobelli J, Spagnolo DV, Tesfai Y, et al. Cutaneous intravascular anaplastic large T-cell lymphoma: a case report and review of the literature. Am J Dermatopathol 2012;34(8):e133–8.

77. Wang L, Li C, Gao T. Cutaneous intravascular anaplastic large cell lymphoma. J Cutan Pathol 2011;38(2):221–6.

78. Geissinger E, Sadler P, Roth S, et al. Disturbed expression of the T-cell receptor/CD3 complex and associated signaling molecules in CD30+ T-cell lymphoproliferations. Haematologica 2010; 95(10):1697–704.

79. Felgar RE, Macon WR, Kinney MC, et al. TIA-1 expression in lymphoid neoplasms. Identification of subsets with cytotoxic T lymphocyte or natural killer cell differentiation. Am J Pathol 1997;150(6): 1893–900.

80. Bijl JJ, Rieger E, van Oostveen JW, et al. HOXC4, HOXC5, and HOXC6 expression in primary cutaneous lymphoid lesions. High expression of HOXC5 in anaplastic large-cell lymphomas. Am J Pathol 1997;151(4):1067–74.

81. Macgrogan G, Vergier B, Dubus P, et al. CD30-positive cutaneous large cell lymphomas. A comparative study of clinicopathologic and molecular features of 16 cases. Am J Clin Pathol 1996;105(4):440–50.

82. DeCoteau JF, Butmarc JR, Kinney MC, et al. The t(2;5) chromosomal translocation is not a common feature of primary cutaneous CD30+ lymphoproliferative disorders: comparison with anaplastic large-cell lymphoma of nodal origin. Blood 1996; 87(8):3437–41.

83. Kadin ME, Pinkus JL, Pinkus GS, et al. Primary cutaneous ALCL with phosphorylated/activated cytoplasmic ALK and novel phenotype: EMA/MUC1+, cutaneous lymphocyte antigen negative. Am J Surg Pathol 2008;32(9):1421–6.

84. Quintanilla-Martinez L, Jansen PM, Kinney MC, et al. Non-mycosis fungoides cutaneous T-cell lymphomas: report of the 2011 Society for Hematopathology/European Association for Haematopathology workshop. Am J Clin Pathol 2013;139(4):491–514.

85. Oschlies I, Lisfeld J, Lamant L, et al. ALK-positive anaplastic large cell lymphoma limited to the skin: clinical, histopathological and molecular analysis of 6 pediatric cases. A report from the ALCL99 study. Haematologica 2013;98(1):50–6.

86. Lamant L, Pileri S, Sabattini E, et al. Cutaneous presentation of ALK-positive anaplastic large cell lymphoma following insect bites: evidence for an association in five cases. Haematologica 2010; 95(3):449–55.

87. Kempf W, Rozati S, Kerl K, et al. Cutaneous peripheral T-cell lymphomas, unspecified/NOS and rare subtypes: a heterogeneous group of challenging cutaneous lymphomas. G Ital Dermatol Venereol 2012;147(6):553–62.

88. van Kester MS, Tensen CP, Vermeer MH, et al. Cutaneous anaplastic large cell lymphoma and peripheral T-cell lymphoma NOS show distinct chromosomal alterations and differential expression of chemokine receptors and apoptosis regulators. J Invest Dermatol 2010;130(2):563–75.

89. Pham-Ledard A, Prochazkova-Carlotti M, Laharanne E, et al. IRF4 gene rearrangements define a subgroup of CD30-positive cutaneous T-cell lymphoma: a study of 54 cases. J Invest Dermatol 2010;130(3):816–25.

90. Benner MF, Ballabio E, van Kester MS, et al. Primary cutaneous anaplastic large cell lymphoma shows a distinct miRNA expression profile and reveals differences from tumor-stage mycosis fungoides. Exp Dermatol 2012;21(8):632–4.

91. Suga H, Sugaya M, Miyagaki T, et al. Differential patterns of CXCR3, CCR3, and CCR10 expression in mycosis fungoides, Sezary syndrome and CD30(+) lymphoproliferative disorders: immunohistochemical study of 43 samples. J Dermatol Sci 2011;64(2):142–4.

92. Carrozza PM, Kempf W, Kazakov DV, et al. A case of Sezary's syndrome associated with granulomatous lesions, myelodysplastic syndrome and transformation into CD30-positive large-cell pleomorphic lymphoma. Br J Dermatol 2002;147(3): 582–6.

93. Baum CL, Stone MS, Liu V. Atypical intravascular CD30+ T-cell proliferation following trauma in a healthy 17-year-old male: first reported case of a potential diagnostic pitfall and literature review. J Cutan Pathol 2009;36(3):350–4.

94. Riveiro-Falkenbach E, Fernandez-Figueras MT, Rodriguez-Peralto JL. Benign atypical intravascular CD30(+) T-cell proliferation: a reactive condition mimicking intravascular lymphoma. Am J Dermatopathol 2013;35(2):143–50.

95. Zizi-Sermpetzoglou A, Petrakopoulou N, Tepelenis N, et al. Intravascular T-cell lymphoma of the vulva, CD30 positive: a case report. Eur J Gynaecol Oncol 2009;30(5):586–8.

96. Benner MF, Willemze R. Bone marrow examination has limited value in the staging of patients with an anaplastic large cell lymphoma first presenting in the skin. Retrospective analysis of 107 patients. Br J Dermatol 2008;159(5):1148–51.

97. Benner MF, Willemze R. Applicability and prognostic value of the new TNM classification system in 135 patients with primary cutaneous anaplastic large cell lymphoma. Arch Dermatol 2009;145(12): 1399–404.

98. Woo DK, Jones CR, Vanoli-Storz MN, et al. Prognostic factors in primary cutaneous anaplastic large cell lymphoma: characterization of clinical subset with worse outcome. Arch Dermatol 2009;145(6): 667–74.

99. Liu HL, Hoppe RT, Kohler S, et al. CD30+ cutaneous lymphoproliferative disorders: the Stanford experience in lymphomatoid papulosis and primary cutaneous anaplastic large cell lymphoma. J Am Acad Dermatol 2003;49(6):1049–58.

100. Ravat FE, Spittle MF, Russell-Jones R. Primary cutaneous T-cell lymphoma occurring after organ transplantation. J Am Acad Dermatol 2006;54(4): 668–75.

101. Seckin D, Barete S, Euvrard S, et al. Primary cutaneous posttransplant lymphoproliferative disorders in solid organ transplant recipients: a multicenter European case series. Am J Transplant 2013; 13(8):2146–53.

102. Benner MF, Jansen PM, Vermeer MH, et al. Prognostic factors in transformed mycosis fungoides:

103. Servitje O, Estrach T, Pujol RM, et al. Primary cutaneous marginal zone B-cell lymphoma: a clinical, histopathological, immunophenotypic and molecular genetic study of 22 cases. Br J Dermatol 2002; 147(6):1147–58.

104. Vempf W, Kazakov DV, Ruetten A, et al. Primary cutanueous follicle center lymphoma with diffuse CD30 expression: a report of 4 cases of a rare variant. J Am Acad Dermatol 2014, in press.

105. Herrera E, Gallardo M, Bosch R, et al. Primary cutaneous CD30 (Ki-1)-positive non-anaplastic B-cell lymphoma. J Cutan Pathol 2002;29(3):181–4.

106. Oguz O, Engin B, Demirkesen C. Primary cutaneous CD30-positive large B-cell lymphoma associated with Epstein-Barr virus. Int J Dermatol 2003;42(9):718–20.

107. Duvic M, Reddy SA, Pinter-Brown L, et al. A phase II study of SGN-30 in cutaneous anaplastic large cell lymphoma and related lymphoproliferative disorders. Clin Cancer Res 2009;15(19): 6217–24.

108. Younes A, Bartlett NL, Leonard JP, et al. Brentuximab vedotin (SGN-35) for relapsed CD30-positive lymphomas. N Engl J Med 2010; 363(19):1812–21.

109. Wasik MA, Jimenez GS, Weisenburger DD. Targeting CD30 in malignant tissues: challenges in detection and clinical applications. Pathobiology 2013; 80(5):252–8.

a retrospective analysis of 100 cases. Blood 2012;119(7):1643–9.

CD30-Negative Cutaneous T-Cell Lymphomas Other than Mycosis Fungoides

Rein Willemze, MD

KEYWORDS

- Cutaneous T-cell lymphoma • Subcutaneous panniculitis–like T-cell lymphoma
- Extranodal NK/T-cell lymphoma, nasal type • Adult T-cell leukemia/lymphoma
- Primary cutaneous peripheral T-cell lymphoma, not otherwise specified
- Primary cutaneous aggressive epidermotropic CD8$^+$ cytotoxic T-cell lymphoma
- Primary cutaneous gamma-delta T-cell lymphoma
- Primary cutaneous CD4-positive small-medium pleomorphic T-cell lymphoma

KEY POINTS

- Histopathologic criteria are insufficient to differentiate between different types of cutaneous T-cell lymphoma (CTCL). Correct classification requires integration of histopathologic findings with clinical data and with the results of immunophenotypic and often genetic data.
- In every patient with a diagnosis of primary cutaneous peripheral T-cell lymphoma, not otherwise specified (PTCL, NOS), the diagnosis of mycosis fungoides (MF) should be ruled out by an accurate clinical history, complete clinical examination, and biopsy of any concurrent eczematous skin lesions.
- The category of non-MF CD30-negative CTCL includes both indolent (subcutaneous panniculitis–like T-cell lymphoma [SPTCL] and primary cutaneous CD4-positive small-medium pleomorphic T-cell lymphoma [PCSM-TCL]) and aggressive entities (extranodal natural killer [NK]/T-cell lymphoma, nasal type; PTCL, NOS; primary cutaneous aggressive epidermotropic CD8$^+$ cytotoxic T-cell lymphoma [CD8$^+$ AECTCL]; and primary cutaneous gamma-delta T-cell lymphoma [PCGD-TCL]).

ABSTRACT

Cutaneous T-cell lymphomas (CTCLs), other than mycosis fungoides/Sézary syndrome and the group of cutaneous CD30$^+$ lymphoproliferative disorders, are rare. These include subcutaneous panniculitis–like T-cell lymphoma (SPTCL); extranodal natural killer/T-cell lymphoma, nasal type; primary cutaneous peripheral T-cell lymphoma, not otherwise specified (PTCL, NOS); and rare subtypes of PTCL, NOS. Apart from SPTCL and primary cutaneous CD4-positive small-medium pleomorphic T-cell lymphoma, these lymphomas have in common aggressive clinical behavior and poor prognosis. Differentiation between these different types of CTCL may be difficult and requires integration of histopathologic findings with clinical data and the results of phenotypic and often molecular genetic studies.

OVERVIEW

The term, *CTCL*, refers to T-cell lymphomas that present in the skin with no evidence of

Conflict of Interest: None declared.
Department of Dermatology, Leiden University Medical Center, B1-Q-93, PO Box 9600, Leiden 2300 RC, The Netherlands
E-mail address: rein.willemze@planet.nl

Surgical Pathology 7 (2014) 229–252
http://dx.doi.org/10.1016/j.path.2014.02.006
1875-9181/14/$ – see front matter © 2014 Elsevier Inc. All rights reserved.

extracutaneous disease at the time of diagnosis. In the World Health Organization–European Organization for Research and Treatment of Cancer (WHO-EORTC) classification for primary cutaneous lymphomas and WHO 2008 classification, 3 major categories of CTCL can be distinguished: (1) the group of classical CTCLs, including MF, variants of MF, and Sézary syndrome; (2) the group of primary cutaneous CD30$^+$ lymphoproliferative disorders (LPDs), including cutaneous anaplastic large cell lymphoma (C-ALCL) and lymphomatoid papulosis (LyP); and (3) a group of rare, often aggressive, cutaneous T/NK-cell lymphomas, including SPTCL; extranodal NK/T-cell lymphoma, nasal type; and PTCL, NOS.[1,2] Because of their characteristic clinicopathologic, phenotypical, and prognostic features, 3 subtypes of PTCL, NOS have been delineated and included as provisional entities in the WHO-EORTC classification. These include CD8$^+$ AECTCL, PCGD-TCL, and PCSM-TCL. In the WHO 2008 classification, these 3 lymphomas have been included in a separate category of primary cutaneous peripheral T-cell lymphoma, rare subtypes, with CD8$^+$ AECTCL and PCSM-TCL as provisional entities. For cases that do not fit into any of these 3 subgroups, the designation, primary cutaneous PTCL, NOS, is maintained.

In the Western world, the first 2 major categories account for approximately 90% of CTCLs. The remaining CTCLs, discussed in this article, account for less than 10% (Table 1). Different distributions have been observed, however, in other parts of the world.[3,4]

Because of overlapping clinicopathologic features, differentiation between these different entities may be difficult. Moreover, distinction from MF may be impossible if detailed clinical information is lacking. Correct diagnosis and classification is only possible if histologic findings are combined with clinical data and the results of extensive phenotypical analysis and molecular genetic studies.

The characteristic clinicopathologic features and differential diagnosis of these uncommon types of CTCL are described.

SUBCUTANEOUS PANNICULITIS–LIKE T-CELL LYMPHOMA

OVERVIEW

SPTCL was originally defined as a cytotoxic T-cell lymphoma, which preferentially infiltrates the subcutaneous tissue, is often complicated by a hemophagocytic syndrome (HPS), has an aggressive clinical course, and should therefore be treated

Table 1
Relative frequency of different types of CTCL in the Western world

WHO-EORTC Classification	Frequency (%)[a]
MF	48
MF variants	
Folliculotropic MF	9
Pagetoid reticulosis	<1
Granulomatous slack skin	<1
Sézary syndrome	3
Adult T-cell leukemia/lymphoma	<1
Primary cutaneous CD30$^+$ LPDs	
C-ALCL	12
LyP	20
SPTCL	1
Extranodal NK/T-cell lymphoma, nasal type	<1
Primary cutaneous peripheral T-cell lymphoma, rare subtypes	
PCGD-TCL	<1
CD8$^+$ AECTCL (provisional)	<1
PCSM-TCL (provisional)	3
PTCL, NOS	3

[a] Based on 2010 patients with a CTCL included in the Dutch Cutaneous Lymphoma Registry between 1986 and 2013.

with aggressive multiagent chemotherapy.[5,6] In past classification schemes, SPTCL included cases of an αβ T-cell phenotype (75%) and cases of a γδ T-cell phenotype (25%).[6,7] More recent studies, however, showed clinical, histologic, and immunophenotypical differences between SPTCL with an αβ T-cell phenotype and SPTCL with a γδ T-cell phenotype, suggesting that these may represent different entities (Table 2).[8,9] In recent classifications, the term, SPTCL, is used only for cases with an αβ T-cell phenotype, whereas cases of expression of γδ T-cell receptor (TCR) are now reclassified as PCGD-TCL.[1,2]

CLINICAL FEATURES

SPTCL occurs in adults as well as young children. Patients generally present with solitary or multiple nodules or deeply seated plaques with a diameter varying between 1 and 20 cm. The skin lesions mainly involve the legs, the arms, the trunk, and less commonly the face and may leave areas of lipoatrophy after disappearance (Fig. 1). Ulceration is

Table 2
Distinguishing features between subcutaneous panniculitis–like T-cell lymphoma and primary cutaneous gamma-delta T-cell lymphoma

	SPTCL	PCGD-TCL
Immunophenotype	TCRβ⁺, CD4⁻, CD8⁺, CD56⁻	TCRγ⁺, CD4⁻, CD8⁻/⁺, CD56⁺/⁻
Architecture	Subcutaneous	Subcutaneous and/or epidermal/dermal
Clinical features	Nodules and plaques; rarely ulceration; association with autoimmune disorders (20%)	Nodules and plaques Ulceration common
HPS	Uncommon (17%)	Common (50%)
5-Year survival (%)	82[a]	11
Treatment	Systemic steroids	Systemic chemotherapy

[a] 5-Year survival: 91% in patients with HPS, 46% in patients with HPS.[9]

uncommon. Systemic symptoms, such as fever, fatigue, and weight loss, and laboratory abnormalities, including cytopenias and elevated liver function tests, are common, but a frank HPS is observed in only 15% of patients.[5,9] Dissemination to extracutaneous sites is rare. Hepatosplenomegaly may be seen but is generally not due to lymphomatous involvement. Up to 20% of patients may have associated autoimmune disease, most commonly systemic lupus erythematosus.[9]

DIAGNOSIS: MICROSCOPIC FEATURES

Histologically, SPTCL reveals subcutaneous infiltrates simulating a lobular panniculitis showing small, medium-sized, or sometimes large pleomorphic T cells with hyperchromatic nuclei and often many macrophages (**Fig. 2**A). The overlying epidermis and dermis are typically uninvolved. Rimming of individual fat cells by neoplastic T cells is a helpful, although not completely specific, diagnostic feature (see **Fig. 2**B). Necrosis, karyorrhexis, cytophagocytosis, and fat necrosis are common findings.[10] In the early stages, the neoplastic infiltrates may lack significant atypia and a heavy inflammatory infiltrate may predominate.[11,12]

DIAGNOSIS: ANCILLARY STUDIES

The neoplastic cells have a mature CD3⁺, CD4⁻, CD8⁺ T-cell phenotype, with expression of cytotoxic proteins (see **Fig. 2**C).[8–10,13] The neoplastic T cells express βF1 but not TCRγ and are negative

Fig. 1. SPTCL. Subcutaneous nodules on the left arm. Ulceration is not present.

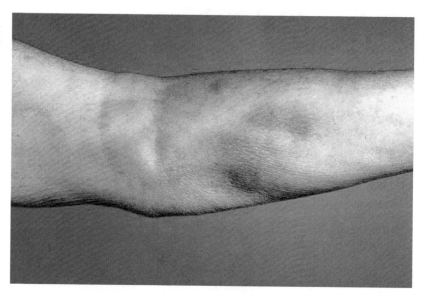

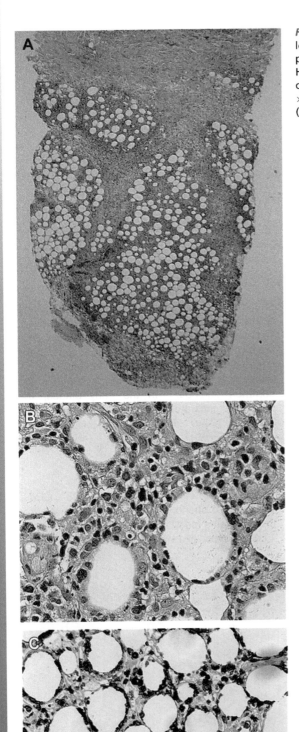

Fig. 2. SPTCL. (*A*) Infiltrates are almost exclusively localized in subcutaneous tissue resembling a lobular panniculitis (HE, original magnification ×25). (*B*) Higher detail showing rimming of individual adipocytes by neoplastic T-cells (HE, original magnification ×480). (*C*) Tumor cells show positive staining for CD8 (original magnification ×480).

for CD56, facilitating differentiation from cutaneous gamma-delta T-cell lymphoma.[9,14] CD30 is rarely, if ever, expressed. The neoplastic T cells show clonal TCR gene rearrangements. Epstein-Barr virus (EBV) is absent.[1]

DIFFERENTIAL DIAGNOSIS

The differential diagnosis of SPTCL includes other types of CTCL with subcutaneous involvement, in particular PCGD-TCL, and lupus panniculitis. In contrast to SPTCL, PCGD-TCL with panniculitis-like features commonly involves not only the subcutis but also the dermis and/or epidermis, either in the same or in other biopsies, and may show ulceration. By definition they have a γδ T-cell phenotype (positive staining for TCRγ/TCRδ, preferably in combination with a negative staining for βF1), are generally negative for both CD4 and CD8, and commonly express CD56 (see **Table 2**). Differentiation is important, because PCGD-TCL with panniculitis-like features generally has a poor prognosis and requires systemic chemotherapy.[9,14]

SPTCL and lupus panniculitis have overlapping clinicopathologic features, making differentiation sometimes extremely difficult.[15,16] The clinical presentation may be identical and several reports describe patients who had both SPTCL and genuine lupus erythematosus.[9,16] As a result, there is controversy whether both conditions may coexist or form a spectrum of disease.[15–17] Histologic features of lupus panniculitis, not or rarely observed in SPTCL, include the presence of interface dermatitis, clusters of B cells (sometimes with formation of germinal centers), and many admixed plasma cells. High proliferation rate and demonstration of clonal TCR gene rearrangements are uncommon in lupus panniculitis and strongly support a diagnosis of SPTCL.

PROGNOSIS

SPTCLs have an excellent prognosis, particularly if not associated with an HPS.[9,10] In a recent EORTC study, patients with and without an associated HPS had 5-year overall survival rates of 46% and 91%, respectively.[9] In SPTCL without associated HPS, systemic steroids or other immunosuppressive agents are recommended, whereas in cases of solitary skin lesions, radiotherapy is advised.[9,10] Only in cases of progressive disease not responding to immunosuppressive therapy and in cases of HPS should multiagent chemotherapy be considered.

EXTRANODAL NK/T-CELL LYMPHOMA, NASAL TYPE

OVERVIEW

Extranodal NK/T-cell lymphoma, nasal type, is an EBV-positive lymphoma of small, medium, or large cells usually with an NK cell or, more rarely a cytotoxic T-cell phenotype. The skin is the second most common site of involvement after the nasal cavity/nasopharynx, and skin involvement may be a primary or secondary manifestation of the disease.[1,2]

CLINICAL FEATURES

Patients are adults, with a predominance of males. This lymphoma is more common in Asia, Central America, and South America. These lymphomas typically present in the nasal cavity or nasopharynx with a midfacial destructive tumor, previously also designated lethal midline granuloma, but may present at other extranodal sites as well.[10,18–21] Patients presenting with skin lesions generally show multiple plaques or tumors, which are preferentially located on the trunk and extremities and commonly, but not invariably, show ulceration (**Fig. 3**).[22] Systemic symptoms, such as fever, malaise, and weight loss, may be present, and some cases are accompanied by HPS.

DIAGNOSIS: MICROSCOPIC FEATURES

These lymphomas show dense infiltrates involving the dermis and often the subcutis. Epidermotropism may be present. Usually there is prominent angiocentricity and angiodestruction, which is often accompanied by extensive tissue necrosis.[19,21] In patients with only nonulcerating skin lesions, however, angiocentricity and angiodestruction may be minimal or even lacking. Extranodal NK/T-cell lymphoma, nasal type, has a broad cytologic spectrum ranging from small to large cells, with most cases consisting of medium-sized cells (**Fig. 4**A). The cells may have irregular or oval nuclei, moderately dense chromatin, and pale cytoplasm. In some cases, a heavy inflammatory infiltrate of small lymphocytes, histiocytes, plasma cells, and eosinophils can be seen.

DIAGNOSIS: ANCILLARY STUDIES

The neoplastic NK cells express CD2, CD56, cytoplasmic CD3ε, and cytotoxic proteins (TIA-1, granzyme B, and perforin) but lack surface CD3 (see **Fig. 4**B,C).[19] In rare CD56-negative cases, detection of EBV by in situ hybridization and expression of cytotoxic proteins are required for diagnosis

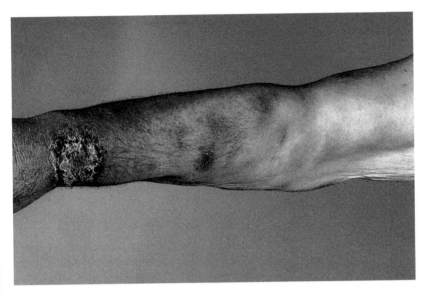

Fig. 3. Extranodal NK/T-cell lymphoma, nasal type. Presentation with generalized plaques and ulcerating tumor on the right wrist.

(see **Fig.** 4D). EBV latent membrane protein (LMP-1) is inconsistently expressed. Most cases have a genuine NK-cell origin with no surface CD3 expression and no TCR expression, together with TCR genes in germline configuration. Some cases, however, may show a true T-cell phenotype with a monoclonal TCR gene rearrangement and surface CD3 expression.[23]

DIFFERENTIAL DIAGNOSIS

Extranodal NK/T-cell lymphoma, nasal type, should be differentiated from other types of aggressive cytotoxic CTCL (PCGD-TCL, CD8[+] AECTCL, and some cases of tumor-stage MF with a cytotoxic phenotype) and from other EBV-associated NK/T-cell LPDs, some of which preferentially affect children.[2] One of these conditions, hydroa vacciniforme–like lymphoma (HVL), is described later. Because extranodal NK/T-cell lymphoma, nasal type, is strongly associated with EBV and most cases have an NK-cell phenotype, demonstration of EBV by EBER in situ hybridization or LMP-1 staining, together with negative staining for T-cell markers and germline configuration of TCR genes, strongly supports a diagnosis of extranodal NK/T-cell lymphoma, nasal type (**Table 3**).

PROGNOSIS

Recent studies indicate that nasal cases have a better prognosis than extranasal cases.[24] Extranodal NK/T-cell lymphoma presenting in the skin is a highly aggressive tumor with a median survival of less than 12 months.[10,20–22] Although

patients presenting with only skin lesions may have a somewhat better prognosis than patients presenting with both cutaneous and extracutaneous disease, the overall prognosis remains poor.[22] CD30[+], CD56[+] cases reported to have a better prognosis most probably have been examples of C-ALCL with coexpression of CD56.[25] In patients with stage I disease, radiotherapy is the first choice of treatment.[26] Cases of more advanced disease show an aggressive clinical behavior and are often resistant to chemotherapy. Recently, an intensive chemotherapy regimen, including steroid (dexamethasone), methotrexate, ifoffamide, L-asparaginase and etoposide (the SMILE regimen), has shown promising effects.[27]

HYDROA VACCINIFORME–LIKE LYMPHOMA

OVERVIEW

HVL is a rare EBV-positive CTCL, clinically resembling hydroa vacciniforme (HV), which is a rare chronic photosensitivity disorder mainly affecting children and characterized by a necrotic papulovesicular eruption with scarring on sun-exposed areas.[28] HVL has been described mainly in children and young adults from Latin American and Asian countries and has been included in the WHO 2008 classification as one of the EBV-positive LPDs of childhood.[2]

CLINICAL FEATURES

Patients present with ulceronecrotic skin lesions associated with blisters, facial edema, and

Fig. 4. Extranodal NK/T-cell lymphoma, nasal type. (*A*) Monotonous infiltration by medium-sized blast cells and extensive karyorrhexis. The tumor cells express CD3ε (HE, original magnification ×480). (*B*) and granzyme B (*C*). In situ hybridization for EBV-encoded RNA is strongly positive (*D*) ([*B–D*], original magnification ×100).

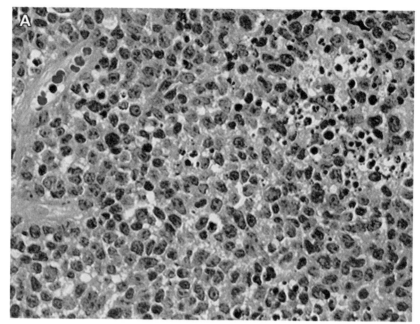

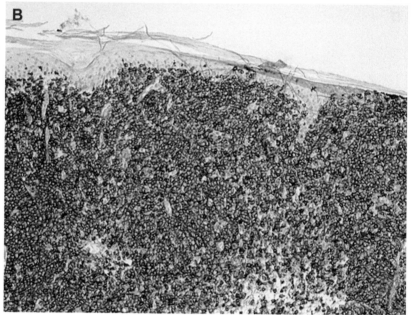

varioliform scars, particularly on the face and extremities.[29,30] Unlike HV, skin lesions in HVL are not limited to sun-exposed areas and do not only appear after sun exposure. Systemic symptoms are frequently observed and include malaise, fever, weight loss, lymphadenopathy, and hepatosplenomegaly. Very similar clinical symptoms may be seen in patients with hypersensitivity to mosquito bites (HMB), a closely related EBV-associated condition.[31]

Fig. 4. (*continued*).

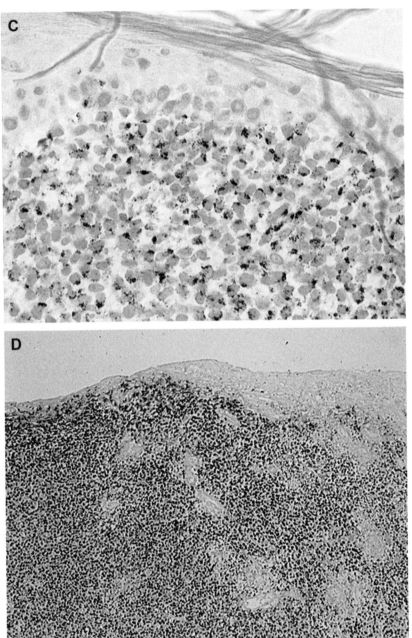

DIAGNOSIS: MICROSCOPIC FEATURES

Histologically, HVL is characterized by the presence of dense lymphoid infiltrates that may extend from the epidermis into the subcutis, showing angiocentricity and angiodestruction, necrosis, and infiltration of adnexal structures. The epidermis is frequently ulcerated. The neoplastic cells are generally small to medium-sized without significant atypia.

Table 3
Distinguishing clinical and immunophenotypic features of different types of CTCL

	Clinical Features	Most Common Phenotype	Cytotoxic Proteins	CD56	Major Lineage	EBV
SPTCL	Subcutaneous nodules and plaques	CD3$^+$, CD4$^-$, CD8$^+$	+	−	αβ T cell	−
Extranodal NK/T-cell lymphoma	(Ulcerating) plaques and tumors	CD3e$^+$, CD4$^-$, CD8$^+$ (surface CD3$^-$)	+	+	NK	+
HVL	Ulceronecrotic skin lesions and varioliform scars, facial edema	CD3$^+$, CD4$^-$, CD8$^+$	+	−	Cytotoxic T cell	+
PCGD-TCL	Ulcerating plaques and tumors	CD3$^+$, CD4$^-$, CD8$^{-/+}$	+	+	γδ T cell	−
CD8$^+$ AECTCL	Ulcerating plaques, nodules and tumors	CD3$^+$, CD4$^-$, CD8$^+$	+	−	αβ T cell	−
PCSM-TCL	Solitary nodule or tumor on the face or upper trunk	CD3$^+$, CD4$^+$, CD8$^-$, PD-1$^+$	−	−	αβ T cell	−
PTCL, NOS	(Ulcerating) plaques and tumors; no prior or concurrent MF	CD3$^+$, CD4$^{+/-}$, CD8$^{-/+}$, CD30$^-$	−/+	−/+	αβ T cell	−
MF	Patches and plaques; (ulcerating) tumors in advanced stage	CD3$^+$, CD4$^+$, CD8$^-$	−/+	−	αβ T cell	−
C-ALCL	Solitary or localized nodules or tumors	CD3$^+$, CD4$^+$, CD8$^-$, CD30$^+$	+/−	−	αβ T cell	−

DIAGNOSIS: ANCILLARY STUDIES

The neoplastic cells most commonly have a CD8$^+$ cytotoxic T-cell phenotype and, less often, an NK-cell phenotype. CD56 is only expressed in cases of an NK-cell phenotype, mainly in patients with HMB.[32] EBV is expressed by all atypical cells, as demonstrated by EBER in situ hybridization. Cases of a cytotoxic T-cell phenotype show clonal TCR gene rearrangements.

DIFFERENTIAL DIAGNOSIS

HV, HMB, and HVL seem to represent different cutaneous manifestations of chronic active EBV infection and have overlapping clinicopathologic features. Distinction between HV and HVL may, therefore, be difficult. Features suggesting a diagnosis of HVL include the presence of skin lesions in non–sun-exposed areas, facial edema, and systemic symptoms as well as detection of clonal TCR gene rearrangements.[30,33] Demonstration of T-cell clonality, however, is not necessarily predictive of an aggressive clinical course.[33]

PROGNOSIS

Most reported cases run an aggressive clinical course and have a poor prognosis, in particular patients presenting with systemic manifestations.[30] Patients may have recurrent skin lesions, however, for many years before progression to systemic lymphoma. Most reported patients have been treated with multiagent chemotherapy, but sustained complete remissions are rarely achieved.[34] In patients with only skin lesions, a conservative approach should be considered.

PRIMARY CUTANEOUS GAMMA-DELTA T-CELL LYMPHOMA

OVERVIEW

PCGD-TCL is a lymphoma composed of a clonal proliferation of mature, activated γδ T cells with a cytotoxic phenotype. This group includes subcutaneous cases previously known as SPTCL with a γδ phenotype.

CLINICAL FEATURES

PCGD-TCL generally presents with disseminated plaques and/or ulceronecrotic nodules or tumors, particularly on the extremities, but other sites may be affected as well (**Fig. 5**).[9,14] Involvement of mucosal and other extranodal sites is frequently observed, but involvement of lymph nodes, spleen, or bone marrow is uncommon.[35] HPS

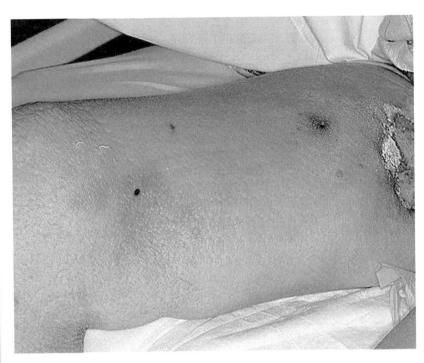

Fig. 5. PCGD-TCL. Nodular and ulcerating skin lesions.

may occur, in particular in patients with panniculitis-like tumors.[9,14]

DIAGNOSIS: MICROSCOPIC FEATURES

In contrast to cases of SPTCL, the neoplastic infiltrates in PCGD-TCL are not confined to the subcutaneous tissue but generally involve the epidermis and/or dermis as well (**Fig. 6**).[9,14] Epidermal infiltration may occur as mild epidermotropism to marked pagetoid reticulosis–like infiltrates, which may be associated with intraepidermal vesiculation and necrosis. Angiocentricity, angiodestruction, and tissue necrosis are common.[9,14,36,37] The neoplastic cells are generally medium to large in size with coarsely clumped chromatin. Large blastic cells with vesicular nuclei and prominent nucleoli are infrequent.

DIAGNOSIS: ANCILLARY STUDIES

The tumor cells characteristically have a TCRγ, βF1−, CD3+, CD2+, CD5−, CD56+ phenotype with strong expression of cytotoxic proteins (**Fig. 7**).[9,14,19,35] Most cases lack both CD4 and CD8, although CD8 may be expressed in some cases. The cells show clonal rearrangement of the TCR gamma gene. EBV is negative.[1]

DIFFERENTIAL DIAGNOSIS

PCGD-TCL should be differentiated from SPTCL, other types of aggressive cytotoxic cutaneous T/NK-cell lymphomas, and tumor-stage MF. Differentiation between these different entities may be extremely difficult and requires integration of clinical, histologic, phenotypical, and molecular genetic data (see **Tables 2** and **3**). Similar to SPTCL, subcutaneous cases of PCGD-TCL may show rimming of fat cells but usually show dermal and/or epidermal involvement as well. The availability of new commercially available TCRγ antibodies has been extremely helpful in differentiating between PCGD-TCL and SPTCL, in particular because the TCRδ antibody used previously on frozen sections is not available anymore. TCRγ expression, however, not only is found in PCGD-TCL but has also been reported in other types of CTCL, including rare cases of otherwise classical MF.[38,39]

PROGNOSIS

PCGD-TCL is resistant to multiagent chemotherapy and has a poor prognosis with a median survival of approximately 15 months.[9,14] Patients with subcutaneous fat involvement tend to have a more unfavorable prognosis than patients with

Fig. 6. PCGD-TCL. High-power view of subcutaneous infiltrate showing rimming of fat cells by neoplastic T cells and extensive karyorrhexis (HE, original magnification ×480).

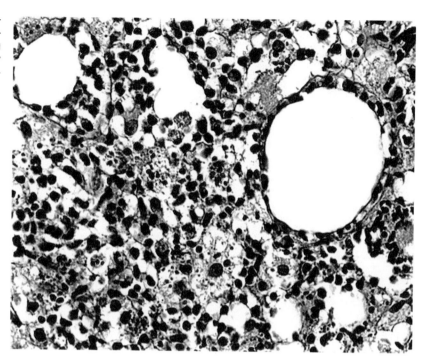

epidermal or dermal disease only.[14] Rare cases of PCGD-TCL with panniculitis-like features, however, following a more indolent clinical course have been reported.[40,41] Patients should be treated with systemic chemotherapy, but the results are often disappointing.[14]

PRIMARY CUTANEOUS AGGRESSIVE EPIDERMOTROPIC CD8-POSITIVE CYTOTOXIC T-CELL LYMPHOMA (PROVISIONAL ENTITY)

OVERVIEW

CD8[+] AECTCLs are characterized by a proliferation of epidermotropic CD8-positive cytotoxic T cells and an aggressive clinical behavior. In the WHO 2008 classification, CD8[+] AECTCL is listed as a provisional entity.[2]

CLINICAL FEATURES

Clinically, these lymphomas show localized or disseminated eruptive papules, nodules, and tumors showing central ulceration and necrosis or by superficial, hyperkeratotic patches and plaques (**Fig. 8**).[13,42] CD8[+] AECTCL may disseminate to visceral sites (lung, testis, central nervous system, and oral mucosa), but lymph nodes are often spared.[42,43]

DIAGNOSIS: MICROSCOPIC FEATURES

The histologic appearance is variable, ranging from a lichenoid pattern with marked, pagetoid epidermotropism and subepidermal edema in early patchlike lesions to diffuse dermal infiltrates in nodular and tumorous lesions (**Fig. 9**). Epidermal necrosis and ulceration, as well as invasion and destruction of adnexal structures, are commonly found.[42,43] Angiocentricity and angioinvasion may be present. Tumor cells are small–medium or medium–large with pleomorphic or blastic nuclei.[1]

DIAGNOSIS: ANCILLARY STUDIES

The tumor cell have a βF1[+], CD3[+], CD8[+], granzyme B[+], perforin[+], TIA-1[+], CD45RA[+/−], CD45RO[−], CD2[−/+], CD4[−], CD5[−], CD7[+/−] phenotype (**Fig. 10**).[10,13,42,43] CD30 is rarely expressed. The neoplastic T cells show clonal TCR gene rearrangements. Specific recurrent genetic abnormalities have not been described. EBV is negative.[1]

DIFFERENTIAL DIAGNOSIS

CD8[+] AECTCL should be differentiated from other types of CTCL expressing a CD8-positive cytotoxic T-cell phenotype (see **Table 3**).[41] Differentiation from SPTCL, early-stage MF, LyP, and pagetoid reticulosis is generally not difficult, in particular when the clinical features are taken

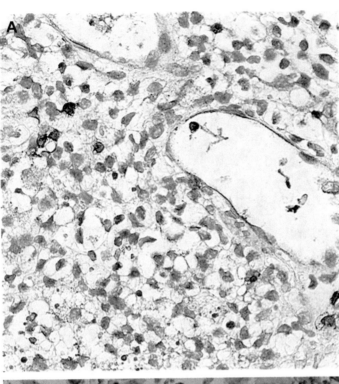

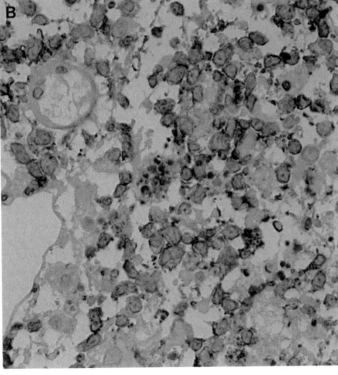

Fig. 7. PCGD-TCL. Neoplastic T-cells do not express βF1 (*A*) but are positive for TCRγ (*B*) ([*A, B*] original magnification ×480).

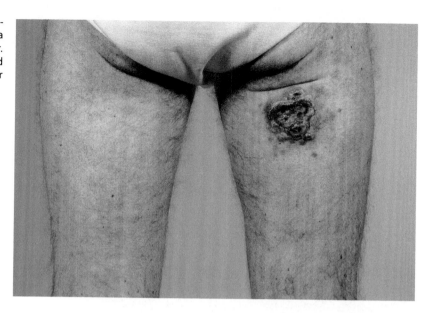

Fig. 8. CD8⁺ AECTCL. Patient presented with a large ulcerating tumor. He died of generalized disease 8 months after diagnosis.

into account. Differentiation from rare cases of CD8⁺ tumor-stage or transformed MF, which may also show ulcerating tumors, may be much more difficult. Clinical information and histologic examination of preceding or concurrent patches or plaques are essential to make a correct diagnosis. CTCLs showing coexpression of CD8 and CD30 most likely belong to the spectrum of primary cutaneous CD30⁺ LPDs, although CD8⁺ AECTCL may occasionally express CD30.

Recent reports describe a new entity designated, *indolent CD8-positive lymphoid proliferation of the ear*.[44] This term has been used for cases presenting with a slowly progressive nodule on the ear (or nose), which combine an indolent clinical course with histologic features suggesting a high-grade malignant lymphoma (**Fig. 11**). These cases show a diffuse proliferation of monomorphous medium-sized cells with a CD3⁺, CD4⁻, CD8⁺, TIA-1⁺, granzyme B⁻, CD30⁻ T-cell phenotype throughout the dermis and subcutis, which is separated from the epidermis by a clear grenz zone (see **Fig. 11B–D**). Loss of pan–T-cell antigens and the presence of clonal TCR gene rearrangements provide further support for the malignant nature of this condition. The proliferation rate, however, is invariably low (<10%). The skin lesions can easily be treated with radiotherapy or excision. Relapses may occur and involve the ears again, but follow-up was uneventful in all patients reported thus far. Recognition that these patients have an indolent clinical behavior, despite an aggressive histology, is important and should prevent unnecessarily aggressive treatment. Recently, similar indolent CD8⁺ cutaneous small

to medium-sized lymphoid proliferations occurring at extrafacial sites have been reported.[45]

PROGNOSIS

These lymphomas often have an aggressive clinical course with a reported median survival of 32 months.[42] Patients should be treated with multiagent chemotherapy, but the results are often disappointing.[1]

PRIMARY CUTANEOUS CD4-POSITIVE SMALL/MEDIUM-SIZED PLEOMORPHIC T-CELL LYMPHOMA (PROVISIONAL ENTITY)

OVERVIEW

In recent classifications, PCSM-TCL is included as a provisional type of CTCL defined by a predominance of small to medium-sized CD4-positive pleomorphic T cells without prior or concurrent patches and plaques typical of MF.[1,2,46]

CLINICAL FEATURES

Characteristically, PCSM-TCL presents with a solitary plaque or tumor, generally on the face, neck, or upper trunk (**Fig. 12**). Less commonly, a presentation with several skin lesions may occur.[46–49]

DIAGNOSIS: MICROSCOPIC FEATURES

These lymphomas show nodular to diffuse dermal infiltrates, which often extend into the subcutaneous fat. Epidermotropism may be present focally. There is a predominance of small/medium-sized

242

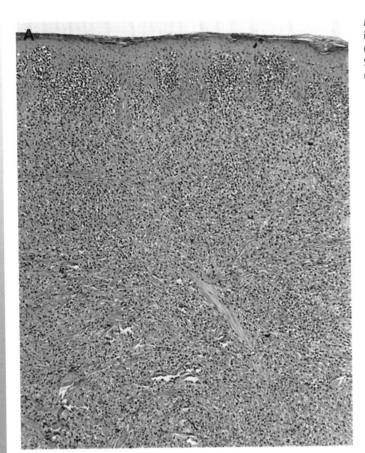

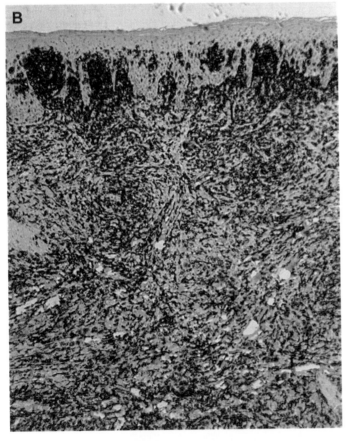

Fig. 9. CD8⁺ AECTCL. (*A*) Diffuse dermal infiltrate with marked epidermotropism (HE, original magnification ×100). (*B*) Strong expression of CD8 (original magnification ×100).

Fig. 10. CD8$^+$ AECTCL. High-power view of infiltrate illustrated in **Fig. 9**. The neoplastic T-cells (*A*) are CD8-positive, (*B*) are CD4-negative, and (*C*) strongly express TIA-1 ([*A–C*], original magnification ×200).

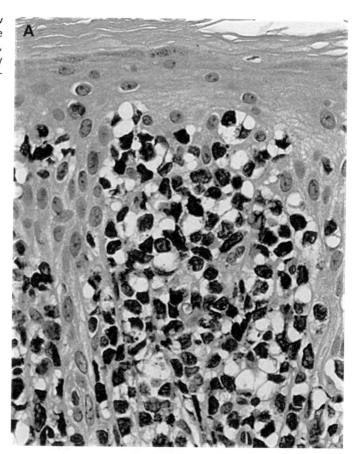

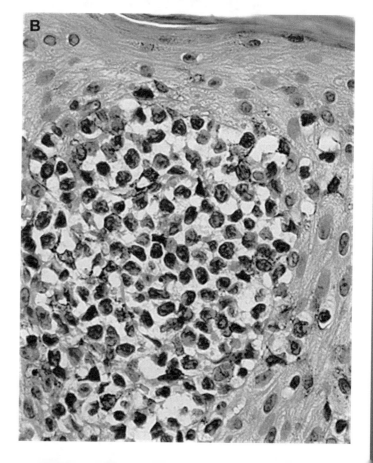

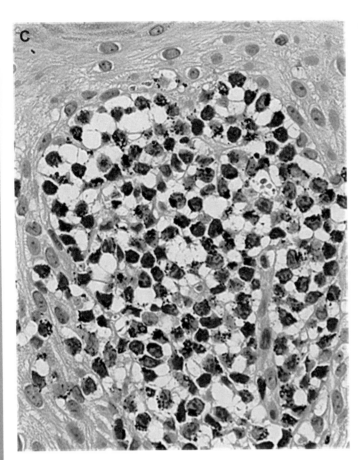

C

Fig. 10. (continued).

pleomorphic T cells. A small proportion (<30%) of large pleomorphic cells may be present (see **Fig. 12**).[50] Almost all cases have a considerable admixture with reactive CD8+ T cells, B cells, plasma cells, and histiocytes, in some cases accompanied by multinucleated giant cells and/or granulomatous changes. Eosinophils are generally few or absent.

DIAGNOSIS: ANCILLARY STUDIES

By definition, these lymphomas have a CD3+, CD4+, CD8−, CD30− phenotype, sometimes with loss of pan–T-cell markers (see **Fig. 12**). The proliferation rate is low, varying between less than 5% and at most 20%. Cytotoxic proteins are not expressed.[46,49] Recent studies showed that the medium-sized to large atypical CD4+ T cells consistently express the follicular helper T-cell markers PD-1, BCL6, and CXCL13, but, unlike angioimmunoblastic T-cell lymphoma, not CD10 (see **Fig. 12**).[41,51,52] EBV is negative. TCR genes are clonally rearranged.[1]

DIFFERENTIAL DIAGNOSIS

The clinical presentation, architecture, and cellular composition of PCSM-TCLs are strikingly similar to those described previously in so-called pseudo–T-cell lymphomas. The relationship between both conditions is a matter of debate. In the 1990s, the term, *pseudo–T-cell lymphoma*, was introduced for lesions with histologic features suggesting a CTCL but a clinical presentation and clinical course more consistent with a benign condition.[53] These pseudo–T-cell lymphomas show the same clinical presentation and clinical course (solitary lesion with an excellent prognosis) and have the same cellular composition (an atypical infiltrate with a predominance of small to medium-sized lymphocytes; variable numbers of medium-sized to large CD3+, CD4+, CD8− T cells expressing PD-1, BCL6, and CXCL13; a considerable admixture with CD8+ T cells, CD20+ B cells, and histiocytes; and low proportion of proliferating cells) as the PCSM-TCL described previously. Demonstration of a T-cell clone and loss of pan–T-cell antigens (except from CD7) are nowadays commonly used

Fig. 11. Indolent CD8-positive lymphoprolifera-tion of the ear. (*A*) Typical clinical presenta-tion with slowly progres-sive skin tumor on the ear (original magnifica-tion ×480). (*B*) Diffuse proliferation of medium-sized pleomorphic cells in the dermis; the atyp-ical cells strongly express CD8 (HE, original magni-fication ×480) (*C*) and TIA-1 (*D*) (original magni-fication ×480).

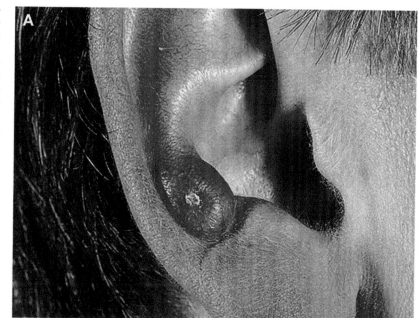

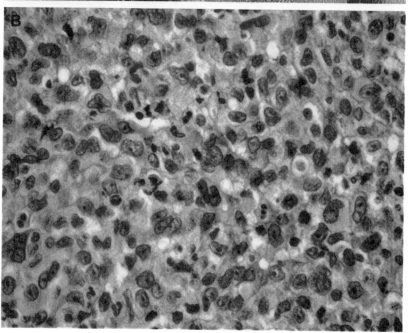

as useful criteria to differentiate PCSM-TCL from pseudo–T-cell lymphomas. With the introduction of more sensitive techniques to demonstrate clon-ality (BIOMED-2 protocols), however, it now seems that most cutaneous pseudo–T-cell lym-phomas contain clonal T cells as well.[52] The over-lapping features between PCSM-TCLs and pseudo–T-cell lymphomas in patients presenting with a solitary lesion are widely recognized. Because differentiating criteria are lacking, *small to medium-sized pleomorphic T-cell nodules of undetermined significance* and *cutaneous CD4+ small–medium T-cell lymphoproliferation* have been suggested as unifying terms for this condi-tion.[41,54] Whichever term is preferred, there is consensus that patients presenting with

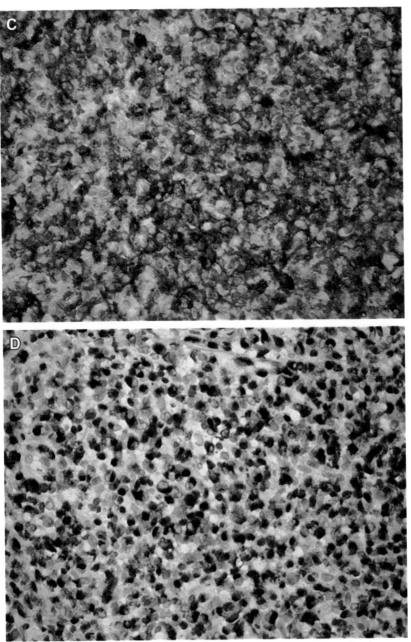

Fig. 11. (continued).

a solitary lesion and the characteristic histologic and immunophenotypical features described in this article (**Table 4**) have an excellent prognosis. Recognition of this entity, separate from other primary cutaneous PTCL, NOS, is important to avoid unnecessarily aggressive treatment of these patients.

PROGNOSIS

Patients presenting with a solitary lesion have an excellent prognosis. A recent study suggested that staging procedures are not required in these patients and that the skin lesions, if not resolved spontaneously after skin biopsy, should be treated

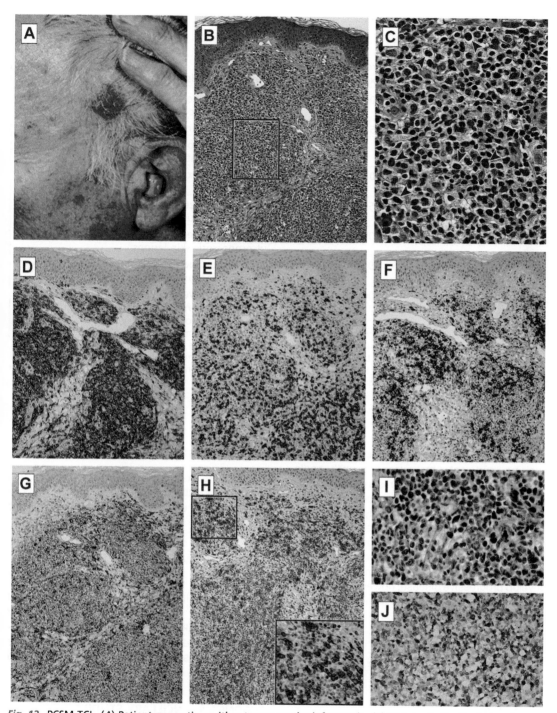

Fig. 12. PCSM-TCL. (*A*) Patient presenting with a tumor on the left temple. (*B*) Histologically, the lesion shows a nonepidermotropic nodular infiltrate throughout the entire dermis. (*C*) At higher magnification, many atypical cells can be seen (indicated by *arrowheads*), which express CD4 (*D*). There is a considerable admixture with reactive CD8+ T-cells (*E*), CD20+ B cells (*F*), and CD68+ histiocytes (*G*). The medium-sized to large atypical T-cells express PD-1 (*H*), BCL6 (*I*), and CXCL13 (*J*). The insert at the bottom of panel H is a higher magnification of the area indicated in the papillary dermis. (*From* Çetinözman F, Jansen PM, Willemze R. Expression of Programmed Death-1 [PD-1] in primary cutaneous CD4-positive small/medium-sized pleomorphic T-cell lymphoma, cutaneous pseudo-T-cell lymphoma, and other types of cutaneous T-cell lymphoma. Am J Surg Pathol 2012;36:112; with permission.)

Table 4
Differential diagnosis of CD8$^+$ CTCL

	Frequency of CD8 Expression (%)	Helpful Distinguishing Features
CD8$^+$ AECTCL	100	Ulcerating plaques, nodules, and tumors; no prior or concurrent eczematous patches/plaques
Early patch/plaque-stage MF	15	Prior or concurrent eczematous patches/plaques[a]
Tumor-stage/transformed MF	5	(Ulcerating) tumors; prior or concurrent eczematous patches/plaques[a]
Pagetoid reticulosis	50	Solitary, slowly expanding plaque; usually on the extremities
C-ALCL	<5	Solitary or localized (ulcerating) tumors; tendency for spontaneous remission[a]
LyP, type D	100	Recurrent, self-healing papular, nodular or small ulceronecrotic skin lesions[a]
SPTCL	>90	Subcutaneous nodules and plaques; no ulceration; no epidermal involvement
Indolent CD8$^+$ lymphoid proliferation of the ear	100	Slowly progressive nodule on ear (or nose); no ulceration; no epidermal involvement; low proliferation rate

[a] No difference in clinical presentation and prognosis between CD8$^+$ and more common CD4$^+$ cases.

Adapted from Quintanilla-Martinez L, Jansen PM, Kinney MC, et al. Non-mycosis fungoides cutaneous T-cell lymphomas: report of the 2011 Society for Hematopathology/European Association for Haematopathology workshop. Am J Clin Pathol 2013;139:507; with permission.

primarily with intralesional steroids or surgical excision and only by exception with radiotherapy.[52] PCSM-TCLs that present with generalized skin lesions and/or do not meet the criteria of the cases described previously are rare and should be fully staged. A recent study suggested that PCSM-TCLs with rapidly growing bulky tumors, a low percentage of admixed CD8$^+$ T cells, and/or a high proliferative fraction are at risk to develop progressive disease; however, this should be confirmed.[48] The optimal treatment in such cases has yet to be defined.

PRIMARY CUTANEOUS PERIPHERAL T-CELL LYMPHOMA, NOT OTHERWISE SPECIFIED

OVERVIEW

The term, *PTCL, NOS*, is used for CTCLs that do not fit into any of the better-defined subtypes of CTCLs, including the 3 rare subtypes of PTCL, NOS, which have been recognized in recent classifications (see **Table 1**). PTCL, NOS can involve the skin primarily or secondarily, but PTCL, NOS presenting with only skin lesions (PTCL, NOS) is uncommon.

CLINICAL FEATURES

Patients are commonly adults who present with solitary or localized, but more frequently generalized, often ulcerating nodules or tumors (**Fig. 13**A).[46,55]

DIAGNOSIS: MICROSCOPIC FEATURES

Histologically, these lymphomas show nodular or diffuse infiltrates with variable numbers of medium-sized to large pleomorphic or immunoblast-like T cells (see **Fig. 13**B). Epidermotropism is generally mild or absent. Large neoplastic cells comprise more than 30% of the infiltrate.[1]

DIAGNOSIS: ANCILLARY STUDIES

Most cases show an aberrant CD4$^+$ T-cell phenotype with variable loss of pan–T-cell antigens. CD30 staining is negative or restricted to few scattered tumor cells. Rare cases may show coexpression of CD56. Expression of cytotoxic proteins is uncommon in CD4$^+$ cases but frequently observed in cases with a CD4$^-$, CD8$^-$ T-cell phenotype.[46]

Fig. 13. PTCL, NOS. (*A*) Patient presenting with generalized nodules and tumors, often with ulceration. (*B*) Diffuse infiltrate of large blast cells, often with prominent nucleoli, expressing a CD3+, CD4−, CD8− T-cell phenotype. A similar histology can be observed in transformed MF. Skin lesions in this patient, however, had started only 3 months previously, and eczematous patches or plaques typical of MF were absent (HE, original magnification ×480).

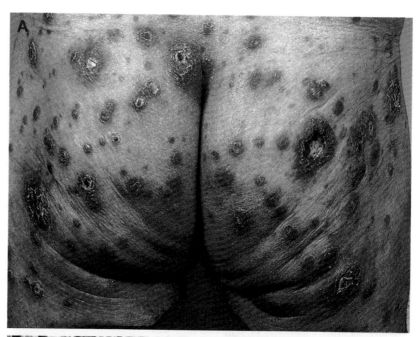

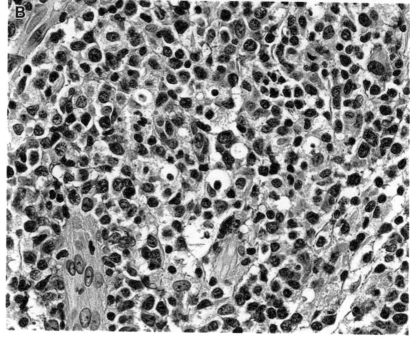

DIFFERENTIAL DIAGNOSIS

Because PTCL, NOS is a diagnosis of exclusion, all other types of CTCL should be ruled out first. In particular, differentiation from transformed MF can be difficult, because the histopathologic features of PTCL, NOS can be identical to those of advanced-stage MF. Clinicopathologic correlation, including an accurate clinical history, complete clinical examination, and biopsy of concurrent eczematous lesions, is required for correct diagnosis. It should be emphasized that patients with MF developing skin lesions or involved lymph nodes with the histologic features of a PTCL, NOS should not be considered to have progressed to a PTCL, NOS and should not be reclassified as such. They simply have tumor-stage MF or nodal involvement by MF. Differentiation is important, because most patients with skin-limited MF should still be treated with skin-directed therapies (eg, radiotherapy), whereas patients with a PTCL, NOS should be treated with multiagent chemotherapy.

PROGNOSIS

The prognosis is generally poor (5-year survival rates less than 20%) and independent of the presence or absence of extracutaneous disease at the time of diagnosis, the extent of skin lesions at presentation, cell size, or expression of CD4[+] or CD8[+] phenotype.[46,47,50,55] Patients are commonly treated with multiagent chemotherapy as with treatment of aggressive T-cell lymphomas.

REFERENCES

1. Willemze R, Jaffe ES, Burg G, et al. WHO-EORTC classification for cutaneous lymphomas. Blood 2005;105:3768–85.
2. Swerdlow A, Campo E, Harris NL, et al. World Health Organization classification of tumours of hematopoietic and lymphoid tissue. Lyon (France): IARC Press; 2008.
3. Tan SH, Sim CS, Ong BH. Cutaneous lymphomas other than mycosis fungoides in Singapore: a clinicopathological analysis using recent classification systems. Br J Dermatol 2003;149:542–53.
4. Park JH, Shin HT, Lee DY, et al. World Health Organization-European Organization for Research and Treatment of Cancer classification of cutaneous lymphoma in Korea: a retrospective study at a single tertiary institution. J Am Acad Dermatol 2012;67:1200–9.
5. Gonzalez CL, Medeiros LJ, Braziel RM, et al. T-cell lymphoma involving subcutaneous tissue. A clinicopathologic entity commonly associated with hemophagocytic syndrome. Am J Surg Pathol 1991;15:17–27.
6. Jaffe ES, Harris NL, Stein H, et al. World Health Organization classification of tumours: pathology and genetics of tumours of hematopoietic and lymphoid tissues. Lyon (France): IARC Press; 2001.
7. Willemze R, Kerl H, Sterry W, et al. EORTC classification for primary cutaneous lymphomas: a proposal from the Cutaneous Lymphoma Study Group of the European Organization for Research and Treatment of Cancer. Blood 1997;90:354–71.
8. Salhany KE, Macon WR, Choi JK, et al. Subcutaneous panniculitis-like T-cell lymphoma: clinicopathologic, immunophenotypic, and genotypic analysis of alpha/beta and gamma/delta subtypes. Am J Surg Pathol 1998;22:881–93.
9. Willemze R, Jansen PM, Cerroni L, et al. Subcutaneous panniculitis-like T-cell lymphoma: definition, classification, and prognostic factors: an EORTC Cutaneous Lymphoma Group Study of 83 cases. Blood 2008;111:838–45.
10. Massone C, Chott A, Metze D, et al. Subcutaneous, blastic natural killer (NK), NK/T-cell, and other cytotoxic lymphomas of the skin: a morphologic, immunophenotypic, and molecular study of 50 patients. Am J Surg Pathol 2004;28:719–35.
11. Hoque SR, Child FJ, Whittaker SJ, et al. Subcutaneous panniculitis-like T-cell lymphoma: a clinicopathological, immunophenotypic and molecular analysis of six patients. Br J Dermatol 2003;148:516–25.
12. Marzano AV, Berti E, Paulli M, et al. Cytophagic histiocytic panniculitis and subcutaneous panniculitis-like T-cell lymphoma: report of 7 cases. Arch Dermatol 2000;136:889–96.
13. Santucci M, Pimpinelli N, Massi D, et al. Cytotoxic/natural killer cell cutaneous lymphomas. Report of EORTC Cutaneous Lymphoma Task Force Workshop. Cancer 2003;97:610–27.
14. Toro JR, Liewehr DJ, Pabby N, et al. Gamma-delta T-cell phenotype is associated with significantly decreased survival in cutaneous T-cell lymphoma. Blood 2003;101:3407–12.
15. Magro CM, Crowson AN, Kovatich AJ, et al. Lupus profundus, indeterminate lymphocytic lobular panniculitis and subcutaneous T-cell lymphoma: a spectrum of subcuticular T-cell lymphoid dyscrasia. J Cutan Pathol 2001;28:235–47.
16. Pincus LB, LeBoit PE, McCalmont TH, et al. Subcutaneous panniculitis-like T-cell lymphoma with overlapping clinicopathologic features of lupus erythematosus: coexistence of 2 entities? Am J Dermatopathol 2009;31:520–6.
17. Magro CM, Crowson AN, Byrd JC, et al. Atypical lymphocytic lobular panniculitis. J Cutan Pathol 2004;31:300–6.
18. Miyamoto T, Yoshino T, Takehisa T, et al. Cutaneous presentation of nasal/nasal type T/NK cell lymphoma: clinicopathological findings of four cases. Br J Dermatol 1998;139:481–7.
19. Jaffe ES, Krenacs L, Raffeld M. Classification of cytotoxic T-cell and natural killer cell lymphomas. Semin Hematol 2003;40:175–84.
20. Cheung MM, Chan JK, Lau WH, et al. Primary non-Hodgkin's lymphoma of the nose and nasopharynx: clinical features, tumor immunophenotype, and treatment outcome in 113 patients. J Clin Oncol 1998;16:70–7.

21. Chan JK, Sin VC, Wong KF, et al. Nonnasal lymphoma expressing the natural killer cell marker CD56: a clinicopathologic study of 49 cases of an uncommon aggressive neoplasm. Blood 1997;89: 4501–13.

22. Bekkenk MW, Jansen PM, Meijer CJ, et al. CD56+ hematological neoplasms presenting in the skin: a retrospective analysis of 23 new cases and 130 cases from the literature. Ann Oncol 2004;15: 1097–108.

23. Pongpruttipan T, Sukpanichnant S, Assanasen T, et al. Extranodal NK/T-cell lymphoma, nasal type, includes cases of natural killer cell and alphabeta, gammadelta, and alphabeta/gammadelta T-cell origin: a comprehensive clinicopathologic and phenotypic study. Am J Surg Pathol 2012;36: 481–99.

24. Au WY, Weisenburger DD, Intragumtornchai T, et al. Clinical differences between nasal and extranasal natural killer/T-cell lymphoma: a study of 136 cases from the International Peripheral T-Cell Lymphoma Project. Blood 2009;113: 3931–7.

25. Mraz-Gernhard S, Natkunam Y, Hoppe RT, et al. Natural killer/natural killer-like T-cell lymphoma, CD56+, presenting in the skin: an increasingly recognized entity with an aggressive course. J Clin Oncol 2001;19:2179–88.

26. Li YX, Yao B, Jin J, et al. Radiotherapy as primary treatment for stage IE and IIE nasal natural killer/ T-cell lymphoma. J Clin Oncol 2006;24:181–9.

27. Yamaguchi M, Kwong YL, Kim WS, et al. Phase II study of SMILE chemotherapy for newly diagnosed stage IV, relapsed, or refractory extranodal natural killer (NK)/T-cell lymphoma, nasal type: the NK-Cell Tumor Study Group study. J Clin Oncol 2011; 29:4410–6.

28. Iwatsuki K, Xu Z, Takata M, et al. The association of latent Epstein-Barr virus infection with hydroa vacciniforme. Br J Dermatol 1999;140:715–21.

29. Barrionuevo C, Anderson VM, Zevallos-Giampietri E, et al. Hydroa-like cutaneous T-cell lymphoma: a clinicopathologic and molecular genetic study of 16 pediatric cases from Peru. Appl Immunohistochem Mol Morphol 2002;10:7–14.

30. Sangueza M, Plaza JA. Hydroa vacciniforme-like cutaneous T-cell lymphoma: clinicopathologic and immunohistochemical study of 12 cases. J Am Acad Dermatol 2013;69:112–9.

31. Kawa K, Okamura T, Yagi K, et al. Mosquito allergy and Epstein-Barr virus-associated T/natural killer-cell lymphoproliferative disease. Blood 2001;98: 3173–4.

32. Hirai Y, Yamamoto T, Kimura H, et al. Hydroa vacciniforme is associated with increased numbers of Epstein-Barr virus-infected gammadeltaT cells. J Invest Dermatol 2012;132:1401–8.

33. Cohen JI, Kimura H, Nakamura S, et al. Epstein-Barr virus-associated lymphoproliferative disease in non-immunocompromised hosts: a status report and summary of an international meeting, 8-9 September 2008. Ann Oncol 2009;20:1472–82.

34. Kimura H, Ito Y, Kawabe S, et al. EBV-associated T/NK-cell lymphoproliferative diseases in nonimmunocompromised hosts: prospective analysis of 108 cases. Blood 2012;119:673–86.

35. De Wolf-Peeters C, Achten R. Gammadelta T-cell lymphomas: a homogeneous entity? Histopathology 2000;36:294–305.

36. Arnulf B, Copie-Bergman C, Delfau-Larue MH, et al. Nonhepatosplenic gammadelta T-cell lymphoma: a subset of cytotoxic lymphomas with mucosal or skin localization. Blood 1998;91: 1723–31.

37. Berti E, Cerri A, Cavicchini S, et al. Primary cutaneous gamma/delta T-cell lymphoma presenting as disseminated pagetoid reticulosis. J Invest Dermatol 1991;96:718–23.

38. Rodriguez-Pinilla SM, Ortiz-Romero PL, Monsalvez V, et al. TCR-gamma expression in primary cutaneous T-cell lymphomas. Am J Surg Pathol 2013;37:375–84.

39. Barzilai A, Goldberg I, Shibi R, et al. Mycosis fungoides expressing gamma/delta T-cell receptors. J Am Acad Dermatol 1996;34:301–2.

40. Magro CM, Wang X. Indolent primary cutaneous gamma/delta T-cell lymphoma localized to the subcutaneous panniculus and its association with atypical lymphocytic lobular panniculitis. Am J Clin Pathol 2012;138:50–6.

41. Quintanilla-Martinez L, Jansen PM, Kinney MC, et al. Non-mycosis fungoides cutaneous T-cell lymphomas: report of the 2011 Society for Hematopathology/European Association for Haematopathology workshop. Am J Clin Pathol 2013;139: 491–514.

42. Berti E, Tomasini D, Vermeer MH, et al. Primary cutaneous CD8-positive epidermotropic cytotoxic T cell lymphomas. A distinct clinicopathological entity with an aggressive clinical behavior. Am J Pathol 1999;155:483–92.

43. Agnarsson BA, Vonderheid EC, Kadin ME. Cutaneous T cell lymphoma with suppressor/cytotoxic (CD8) phenotype: identification of rapidly progressive and chronic subtypes. J Am Acad Dermatol 1990;22:569–77.

44. Petrella T, Maubec E, Cornillet-Lefebvre P, et al. Indolent CD8-positive lymphoid proliferation of the ear: a distinct primary cutaneous T-cell lymphoma? Am J Surg Pathol 2007;31:1887–92.

45. Kempf W, Kazakov DV, Cozzio A, et al. Primary cutaneous CD8(+) small- to medium-sized lymphoproliferative disorder in extrafacial sites: clinicopathologic features and concept on

their classification. Am J Dermatopathol 2013;35: 159–66.

46. Bekkenk MW, Vermeer MH, Jansen PM, et al. Peripheral T-cell lymphomas unspecified presenting in the skin: analysis of prognostic factors in a group of 82 patients. Blood 2003;102:2213–9.

47. Fink-Puches R, Zenahlik P, Back B, et al. Primary cutaneous lymphomas: applicability of current classification schemes (European Organization for Research and Treatment of Cancer, World Health Organization) based on clinicopathologic features observed in a large group of patients. Blood 2002;99:800–5.

48. Garcia-Herrera A, Colomo L, Camos M, et al. Primary cutaneous small/medium CD4+ T-Cell lymphomas: a heterogeneous group of tumors with different clinicopathologic features and outcome. J Clin Oncol 2008;26(20):3364–71.

49. Grogg KL, Jung S, Erickson LA, et al. Primary cutaneous CD4-positive small/medium-sized pleomorphic T-cell lymphoma: a clonal T-cell lymphoproliferative disorder with indolent behavior. Mod Pathol 2008;21:708–15.

50. Beljaards RC, Meijer CJ, Van der Putte SC, et al. Primary cutaneous T-cell lymphoma: clinicopathological features and prognostic parameters of 35 cases other than mycosis fungoides and CD30-positive large cell lymphoma. J Pathol 1994;172:53–60.

51. Rodriguez Pinilla SM, Roncador G, Rodriguez-Peralto JL, et al. Primary cutaneous CD4+ small/medium-sized pleomorphic T-cell lymphoma expresses follicular T-cell markers. Am J Surg Pathol 2009;33:81–90.

52. Cetinozman F, Jansen PM, Willemze R. Expression of programmed death-1 in primary cutaneous CD4-positive small/medium-sized pleomorphic T-cell lymphoma, cutaneous pseudo-T-cell lymphoma, and other types of cutaneous T-cell lymphoma. Am J Surg Pathol 2012;36:109–16.

53. Rijlaarsdam JU, Scheffer E, Meijer CJ, et al. Cutaneous pseudo-T-cell lymphomas. A clinicopathologic study of 20 patients. Cancer 1992;69:717–24.

54. Beltraminelli H, Leinweber B, Kerl H, et al. Primary cutaneous CD4+ small-/medium-sized pleomorphic T-cell lymphoma: a cutaneous nodular proliferation of pleomorphic T lymphocytes of undetermined significance? A study of 136 cases. Am J Dermatopathol 2009;31:317–22.

55. Grange F, Hedelin G, Joly P, et al. Prognostic factors in primary cutaneous lymphomas other than mycosis fungoides and the Sezary syndrome. The French Study Group on Cutaneous Lymphomas. Blood 1999;93:3637–42.

Primary Cutaneous B-Cell Lymphomas

Uma Sundram, MD, PhD[a,b],*

KEYWORDS

- Lymphoma • B cell • Marginal zone lymphoma • Follicle center lymphoma
- Diffuse large B-cell lymphoma • Leg type

ABSTRACT

B-cell lymphomas occurring in the skin often tend to be of systemic origin with secondary cutaneous involvement. Primary cutaneous B-cell lymphomas tend to be indolent disorders, with the exception of primary cutaneous diffuse large B-cell lymphoma–leg type (PCDLBCL-LT). In indolent conditions, the distinction between cutaneous lymphoma and cutaneous lymphoid hyperplasia can be difficult. Integration of all available information, including the clinical setting, is crucial to arriving at the appropriate diagnosis. In this review, we cover the diagnostic approaches to primary cutaneous marginal zone lymphoma, primary cutaneous follicle center lymphoma, and PCDLBCL-LT, and discuss their differential diagnosis.

OVERVIEW

The diagnosis of cutaneous lymphomas in general can be challenging, as these are rare lesions. In particular, primary cutaneous B-cell lymphomas (PCBCLs) can be difficult because the distinction between low-grade primary cutaneous lymphomas and cutaneous lymphoid hyperplasia is not morphologically clear cut. In addition, diffuse variants of primary cutaneous follicle center lymphoma (PCFCL) (that usually demonstrates indolent behavior) can show significant overlap with more aggressive lymphomas, such as primary cutaneous diffuse large B-cell lymphoma–leg type (PCDLBCL-LT). This review is focused on the features of B-cell lymphomas that are truly primary to the skin.

In the 2008 World Health Organization classification of lymphomas, PCFCLs and PCDLBCL-LT have only recently been recognized as entities distinct from their systemic counterparts. This is an important development, as it represents acknowledgment by all physicians involved in the care of these patients that these tumors may represent a completely different group of entities that may require a different pathologic workup and clinical approach than systemic counterparts. Interestingly, primary cutaneous marginal zone lymphoma (PCMZL) is still considered part of the spectrum of extranodal marginal zone lymphoma of mucosa-associated lymphoid tissue (MALT lymphoma), although many features of skin marginal zone lymphomas are quite distinct from gastrointestinal and salivary gland marginal zone lymphomas.

Systemic B-cell lymphomas, whether composed of small or large cells, can show significant overlap with PCBCLs. These include extranodal marginal zone lymphoma, small lymphocytic lymphoma/chronic lymphocytic leukemia (SLL/CLL), and mantle-cell lymphoma (MCL) for the small-cell category of B-cell lymphomas. In the group composed of large B cells, systemic follicular lymphoma is part of the differential, as well as lymphomatoid granulomatosis, cutaneous Epstein-Barr virus (EBV)+ diffuse large B-cell lymphoma (DLBCL) of the elderly (which often presents with concurrent systemic involvement), and T-cell and histiocyte-rich large B-cell lymphoma. If the infiltrate is composed primarily of plasma cells

---

Disclosure Statement: There are no actual or potential conflicts of interest.
[a] Department of Pathology, Stanford Hospital and Clinics, 300 Pasteur Drive Room H2117, Stanford, CA 94305, USA; [b] Department of Dermatology, Stanford Hospital and Clinics, 450 Broadway, Pavilion B 4th Floor, Redwood City, CA 94063, USA
* Department of Dermatology, Stanford Hospital and Clinics, 450 Broadway, Pavilion B 4th Floor, Redwood City, CA 94063.
E-mail address: sundram@stanford.edu

and/or has a concurrent deposition of amyloid, multiple myeloma must enter into the differential. It is therefore essential that all PCBCLs undergo a complete clinical staging workup, which includes imaging studies, blood work, and potentially bone marrow biopsies, if clinically applicable.

PCMZL

OVERVIEW/DEFINITION

PCMZL is a heterogeneous proliferation of marginal zone cells (centrocytelike cells), monocytoid-like B cells, small lymphocytes, and plasma cells.[1] The histologic findings are similar but not identical to entities found in the gastrointestinal tract, salivary gland, and lymph node.[1,2] The 2008 classification of the World Health Organization recently recognized PCMZL as part of so-called MALT lymphomas, but it is important to recognize that many differences exist between other entities of MALT lymphoma and lesions in the skin. For example, although gastric MALT lymphomas have been shown repeatedly to be associated with Helicobacter pylori,[3] only a minority of PCMZL cases have been shown to be associated with Borrelia burgdorferi; this association appears to be present in both endemic and nonendemic areas.[2,4] However, other studies have shown no association between Borrelia burgdorferi and the development of PCMZL.[2] In addition, several terms have been previously used to describe entities that now reside within the category of PCMZL, including so-called cutaneous immunocytoma (cutaneous lymphoplasmacytic lymphoma)[5–7] and cutaneous plasmacytoma.[1,2] These are now considered variants of PCMZL. Lymphoplasmacytic PCMZL is often associated with Borrelia burgdorferi and is common in endemic areas.[2]

CLINICAL FEATURES

Although this disorder can affect all ages, patients are typically younger and a male predominance has been reported.[2] PCMZL, conventional variant, and PCMZL, plasmacytic variant, both have similar clinical presentations. The trunk and extremities are often affected and the head and neck are usually spared sites (**Fig. 1**). The lesions can be solitary or multiple (multifocal disease being more common), and are often reddish purple infiltrated plaques, papules, or nodules. In the lymphoplasmacytic variant, the patients appear to be older and the lower extremities are often affected.[2]

DIAGNOSIS: MICROSCOPIC FEATURES

In conventional PCMZL, on low-power examination the lymphocytic infiltrate can have a nodular or diffuse architecture (**Box 1**). There is usually a Grenz zone and the epidermis is spared; however, rarely epidermotropism has been reported (**Fig. 2**).[8] The infiltrate is heterogeneous,

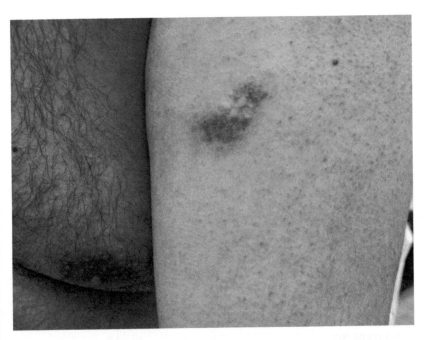

Fig. 1. PCMZL. Two erythematous papulonodules are seen on the upper arm of a 47-year-old man. (*Courtesy of* Youn Kim, MD, Stanford University, Stanford, CA.)

composed of so-called marginal zone cells (centrocytelike cells), small lymphocytes, monocytoidlike B cells, rare large centroblasts, and varying number of plasma cells, histiocytes, and eosinophils (**Figs. 3** and **4**). Centrocytelike cells are small lymphocytes with irregular nuclear outlines, inconspicuous nucleoli, and a fair amount of amphophilic cytoplasm. Monocytoidlike B cells are small lymphocytes with round dark nuclei, inconspicuous nucleoli, and clear or pale-staining cytoplasm. Rare centroblasts, characterized by enlarged irregular nuclei, vesicular chromatin, and prominent nucleoli, are present, as are lymphoplasmacytoid cells, which are ovoid lymphocytes with an eccentrically placed nucleus (**Fig. 5**). Plasma cells often populate the papillary dermis, and if nodules are present, they may be

surrounded by plasma cells (**Fig. 6**). Both superficial and deep infiltrates can be present, and the deep infiltrate can extend into the fat; however, a "top-heavy" infiltrate cannot be dismissed as a reactive process. The infiltrate is often perivascular and periadnexal, but true lymphoepithelial lesions are only rarely present in PCMZL.[9] Less commonly, the neoplastic cells of PCMZL can surround and partially overrun reactive lymphoid follicles with intact or fragmented germinal centers; morphologically, these cases can be difficult to distinguish from cutaneous B-cell–rich lymphoid hyperplasia (CLH-B) and PCFCL. In the lymphoplasmacytic variant, most of the lesional cells are lymphoplasmacytoid cells and plasma cells with few, if any, monocytoid cells. A heterogeneous inflammatory background is not seen and eosinophils and histiocytes are not prominent. Dutcher bodies are often seen, and reactive germinal centers are rare.[2] In the plasmacytic variant, the infiltrate is sheetlike and composed primarily of plasma cells with rare lymphocytes. An inflammatory background is not seen.

DIAGNOSIS: ANCILLARY STUDIES

On immunophenotyping of both the conventional and lymphoplasmacytic variants, the lesional cells (marginal zone cells, small lymphocytes, monocytoidlike B cells, and centroblasts) express CD20 and CD79a, and the plasma cells express CD138 and CD79a (but not CD20) (**Fig. 7**). In a diffuse infiltrate, "sheets" of CD20 and CD79a expressing lymphocytes essentially denotes lymphoma. Often, the CD79a stain highlights more of the infiltrate than the CD20 stain does, as CD79a marks all members of the B-cell ontogeny, including plasma cells (**Fig. 8A**). Both markers should be performed to evaluate the infiltrate in its entirety. In nodular infiltrates, a more extensive panel may need to be performed to assess the infiltrate. Unlike gastric MZL, PCMZL does not express CD5[10] or CD43,[11] although rarely it can express CD23 (see **Fig. 8B**).[12] CD10 and bcl-6 are uniformly negative, as these are germinal center markers. CD21 can help highlight residual germinal centers and cells expressing germinal center markers should be confined to these areas. If a "germinal center–like" area is noted that contains cells expressing CD20 but not bcl-6, this may represent a lesion of PCMZL with overrun residual follicles. The bcl-2 is uniformly positive except within normal germinal centers; however, the ubiquitous nature of bcl-2 expression limits the usefulness of this marker in the diagnosis. Likewise, the proliferation marker Ki67 or mib-1 cannot distinguish between proliferating neoplastic and reactive

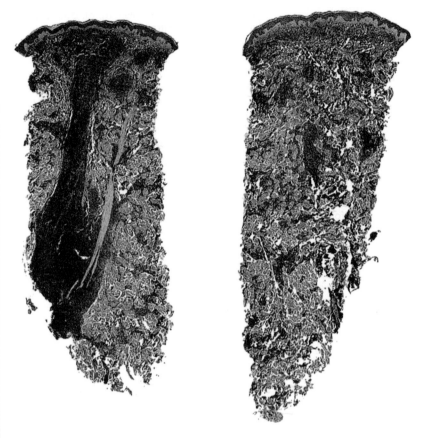

Fig. 2. PCMZL. There is a superficial and deep infiltrate of lymphocytes and plasma cells involving the dermis; a columnar arrangement of cells is seen within the dermis around the remnants of a hair follicle (hematoxylin and eosin [H&E], original magnification ×1).

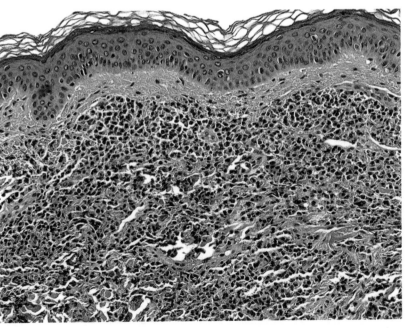

Fig. 3. PCMZL. A dense infiltrate of lymphocytes and plasma cells extends to the papillary dermis and a collection of plasma cells is noted immediately below the epidermis. A Grenz zone is present (H&E, original magnification ×20).

Fig. 4. PCMZL. Plasma cells and marginal zone cells aggregate adjacent to an arrector pili muscle; plasma cells often populate the periphery of nodules in PCMZL (H&E, original magnification ×10).

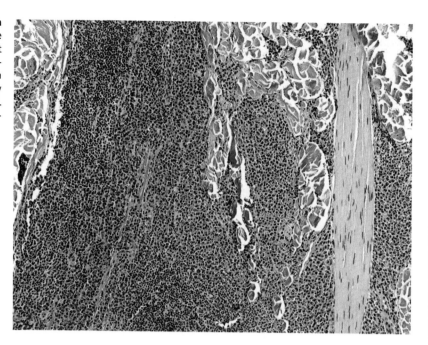

lymphocytes and is of limited utility in the workup of PCMZL. Analysis of expression of kappa and lambda light chains, either by protein staining (immunohistochemistry) or by in situ hybridization (analysis of mRNA expression) is crucial to the diagnosis of PCMZL (**Fig. 9**). Light chain restriction has been reported in up to 93% of PCMZLs.[13] When protein staining is used, the protein can be seen within the cytoplasm placed in an eccentric manner. Examination of light chain restriction via protein staining can be a challenge, as significant amounts of soluble protein are often seen in the

Fig. 5. PCMZL. Higher-power view demonstrates the presence of marginal zone cells, centroblasts, and rare immunoblasts (H&E, original magnification ×40).

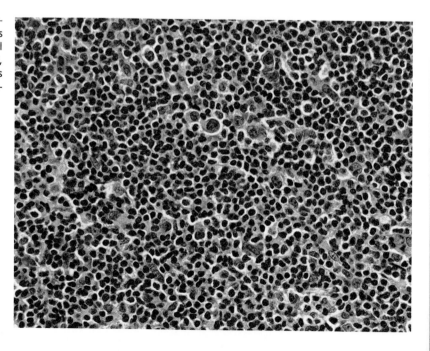

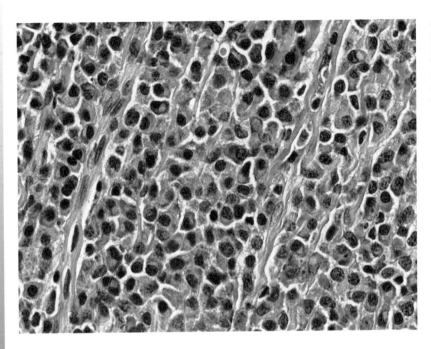

Fig. 6. PCMZL. Higher-power view of the plasma cells of PCMZL, which do not appear morphologically atypical (H&E, original magnification ×60).

surrounding dermal collagen. For this reason, in situ hybridization techniques are often used and have been found to be a more sensitive test for clonality.[2,14] Interestingly, clusters of plasma-cytoid dendritic cells have been found in cases of PCMZL, and these cells express CD123.[15]

Although CLH-B was also demonstrated to have similar clusters of CD123, they were rare in PCFCL, and could be a useful tool in distinguishing between PCMZL and PCFCL. The lesional cells in the plasmacytic variant primarily express CD138 and CD79a, with dim to no

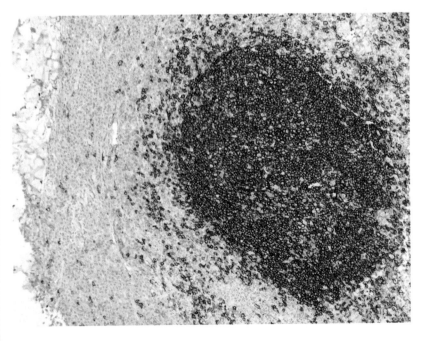

Fig. 7. PCMZL. CD20 highlights the lymphocytes within a nodule of marginal zone lymphoma but the plasma cells are negative (original magnification ×20).

Fig. 8. (A, B) PCMZL. CD79a highlights both the marginal zone cells (weakly) and the plasma cells (strongly) (A). The intervening T cells are negative for this marker (B). (A, CD79a; B, CD3; original magnification ×20 each).

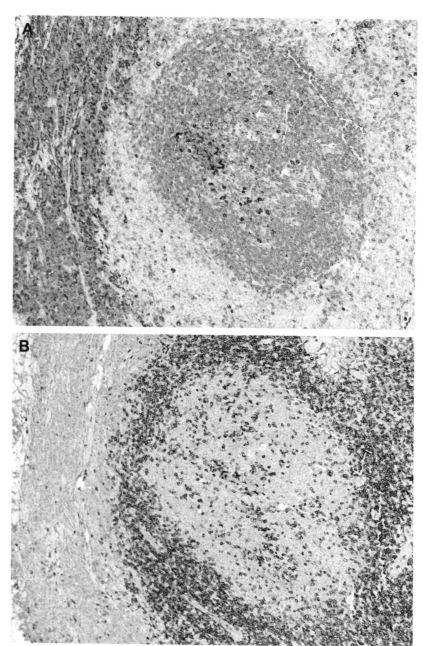

CD20 expression. Light chain expression is easily demonstrated in most cases.

IGH and *IGK* clonality assays are an important aspect for confirming the diagnosis of PCMZL (all variants), especially in ambiguous cases in which the infiltrate is composed of nodules with few plasma cells, reactive cells outnumber neoplastic cells, and light chain restriction cannot be demonstrated. In a recent study of PCBCLs, 12 (80%) of 15 known cases of PCMZL demonstrated the presence of a clone, in comparison with 1 of 23 cases of patients with benign infiltrates.[16] In addition, if more than one lesion is present, testing of both lesions for clones demonstrated the presence of matching clones in 8 (67%) of 12 cases of PCMZL.[17] This finding is not observed in reactive infiltrates. Interestingly, nonmatching clones at disparate skin sites may be present in bona fide cases of lymphoma.

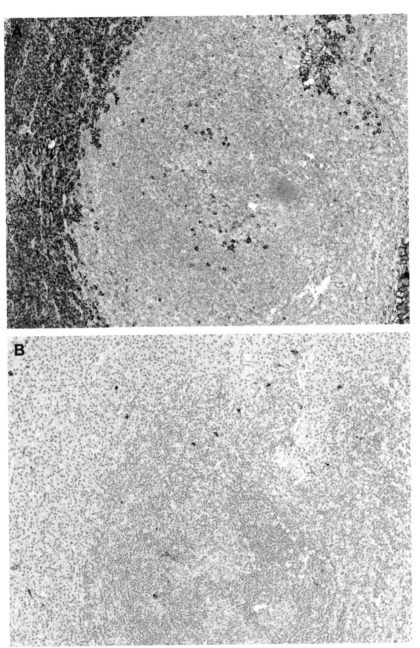

Translocations involving *IGH* and *MALT1* have been described in a subset of PCMZLs, as well as t(3;14)(p14;q32), involving *IGH* and *FOXP1*.[2] Trisomies 3 and 8 have likewise been described in a subset of cases.[1] The t(11;18) translocation is not commonly found in PCMZL.[18,19] Aberrant nuclear bcl-10 has been described, however, and has been thought to be linked to the development of extracutaneous disease.[18]

DIFFERENTIAL DIAGNOSIS

The main differential diagnostic considerations for the conventional variant include CLH-B, low-grade B-cell lymphomas, such as PCFCL, and small B-cell lymphomas/leukemias, such as MCL, and SLL/CLL (**Table 1**).[20] Unlike CLH-B, PCMZL has a predominance of pale-staining marginal zone cells that show extensive encroachment

Table 1
Pathologic features that distinguish between PCMZL, PCFCL, and morphologic mimics

	PCMZL	CLH-B	PCFCL	MCL	SLL/CLL
Neoplastic germinal centers	No	No	Yes	No	No
Monocytoidlike B cells and plasma cells	Yes	No	No	No	Yes[13]
Perivascular and periadnexal accentuation	Yes	Yes, sometimes	No	No	Yes[13]
Germinal center markers are expressed (bcl-6, HGAL, LMO2)	No	No	Yes	No	No
Cyclin D1 (bcl-1) is expressed	No	No	No	Yes	No
CD5 is expressed	No	No	No	Yes	Yes
Light chain restriction	Yes	No	Yes, on flow cytometry and in frozen sections	Yes[1]	Yes[13,20]
Positive IgH/IgK clonality assays	Yes[16,17]	No	Yes	Yes[1]	Yes[1]

Abbreviations: CLH-B, B-cell–rich cutaneous lymphoid hyperplasia; Ig, immunoglobulin; MCL, mantle cell lymphoma; PCFCL, primary cutaneous follicle center lymphoma; PCMZL, primary cutaneous marginal zone lymphoma; SLL/CLL, small lymphocytic lymphoma/chronic lymphocytic leukemia.

into reactive lymphoid follicles (**Figs. 10–13**). A deeply placed infiltrate with extension into fat is more suspicious for lymphoma than for CLH-B. Immunohistochemical findings can be extremely useful; diffuse sheets of CD20+ and CD79a+ cells are confirmatory of lymphoma. Light chain restriction is also a useful feature: kappa-restricted infiltrates contain a greater than 3:1 ratio of kappa to lambda-expressing cells, and lambda-restricted infiltrates contain a greater than 1:1 ratio of lambda to kappa-expressing cells. In cases that do not demonstrate either of these features, clonality assays can be helpful, as a high percentage of PCMZLs are positive for *IGH* and/or *IGK* clones when BIOMED-2 primers and protocols are used with formalin-fixed paraffin-embedded tissues.[16,17] Although only a small number of cases of cutaneous lymphoid hyperplasia were studied in the reports by Morales and colleagues[16] and Fujiwara and colleagues,[17] very few cases demonstrated positive clones using this methodology. Another important member of the differential

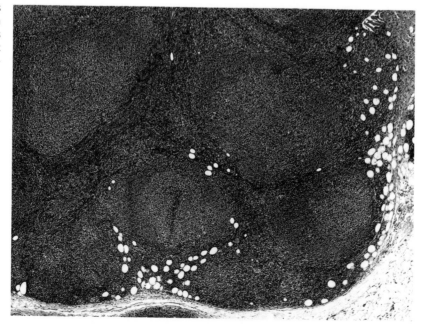

Fig. 10. CLH. Numerous reactive follicles are seen within the deep dermis and subcutaneous fat (H&E, original magnification ×10).

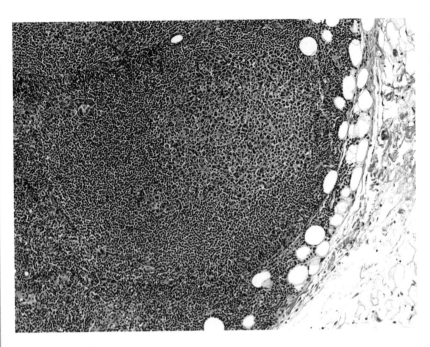

Fig. 11. CLH. Higher-power view of a reactive follicle demonstrates an intact, polarized mantle zone (H&E, original magnification ×20).

diagnosis is low-grade PCFCL; the distinction between these cases and those of nodular PCMZL can be difficult, especially when the latter colonizes preexisting lymphoid follicles. Morphologically, however, the cells within the germinal center should be neoplastic in PCFCL and reactive in PCMZL. One should see small to medium-sized cells with irregularly shaped nuclei (centrocytes) admixed with larger cleaved cells (centroblasts) within the germinal centers in PCFCL. Staining with Ki67 and mib-1 may be useful in this regard: the proliferation rate in a reactive germinal center should be high (more than 90%), whereas that in a reactive germinal center should be low (less than 50%).[21] In addition, replacement of a germinal center–like area with cells that express bcl-2 but not bcl-6 should be a clue to the diagnosis of PCMZL.[22] The lesional cells of PCFCL

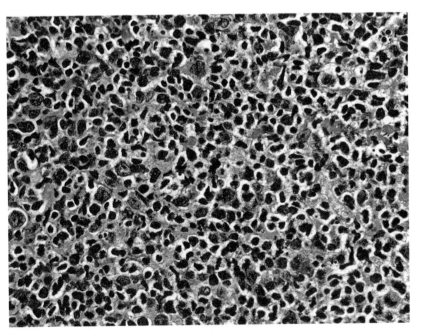

Fig. 12. CLH. Higher-power view of a reactive follicle demonstrates admixture of small and large cells within the germinal center; the large cells are noncleaved (H&E, original magnification ×40).

Fig. 13. CLH. Higher-power view of a reactive follicle demonstrates light staining of the germinal center cells and dark staining of the mantle zone cells by a marker for CD20 (original magnification ×40).

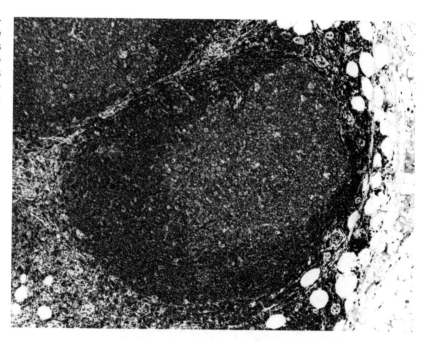

should express germinal center markers. Both entities will show association with CD21 expressing follicular dendritic cell networks. The cells of MCL (secondary cutaneous involvement by systemic MCL) are more angulated and associated with pink histiocytes. They should express CD5 and cyclin-D1 (bcl-1). Finally, it can be challenging to distinguish between SLL/CLL with secondary cutaneous involvement and PCMZL.[13] Both can demonstrate a nodular or diffuse growth pattern, perivascular and periadnexal accentuation of lymphocytes, numerous plasma cells, monocytoidlike B cells, and light chain restriction (**Figs. 14–19**).[13,20] To ensure that SLL/CLL is not missed (especially as skin lesions may be the first clue to a diagnosis of SLL/CLL), CD79a, CD5, CD43, and CD23 should be routinely included in a panel to work up cases of PCMZL.[13]

The cells of extranodal MZL can be identical to PCMZL, conventional variant, but they often express CD43, unlike conventional PCMZL. Expression of CD43 should prompt a workup for systemic disease. In addition, both the lymphoplasmacytic and plasmacytic variants should prompt full staging workups, as they can represent secondary cutaneous involvement by systemic disease. In the case of lymphoplasmacytic PCMZL, Waldenstrom macroglobulinemia is an important differential diagnostic consideration, as this entity has bone marrow involvement and an immunoglobulin (Ig)M monoclonal gammapathy; the lesional cells of this entity show overlap histologically and immunophenotypically with PCMZL. In the case of

the plasmacytic variant, secondary cutaneous involvement by multiple myeloma is always a possibility, and should be excluded clinically. Cases of secondary cutaneous involvement by multiple myeloma often demonstrate atypical plasma cells and deposition of interstitial and perivascular amyloid, which can be a clue to the systemic nature of the disease.[2] Another differential diagnostic consideration includes cutaneous plasmacytosis, a recently described entity that affects Asian individuals and consists of red-brown plaques and nodules on the trunk.[23] Lymphadenopathy and hypergammaglobulinemia may be present. On histology, the skin is involved by a diffuse infiltrate of mature plasma cells, but light chain restriction and cellular atypia are absent. The presence of systemic symptoms excludes PCMZL, and the clinical setting may help in arriving at the appropriate diagnosis for these patients, as extranodal MZL may have similar histologic features. Castleman disease (CD) involving the skin is another potential differential diagnostic partner.[24] CD involving the skin shows all of the features of nodal CD, including an atrophic germinal center without tangible body macrophages, an expanded marginal zone, "onion skin" arrangement of the mantle zone lymphocytes, hyalinized sclerotic collagen fascicles, and a tight/concentric follicular dendritic cell network.[24] The presence of concomitant nodal CD should help eliminate PCMZL. Finally, it is important to note that secondary cutaneous involvement by systemic MZL can show identical histopathologic,

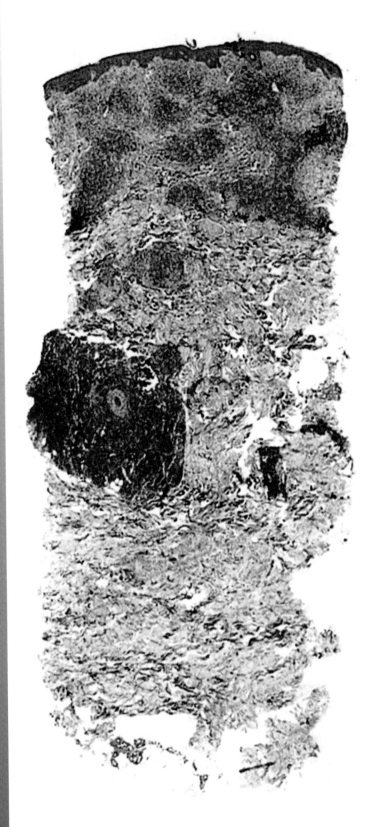

Fig. 14. Cutaneous involvement by CLL. There is a superficial and deep infiltrate of lymphocytes and plasma cells involving the dermis, with a portion of the infiltrate surrounding a hair follicle (H&E, original magnification ×1).

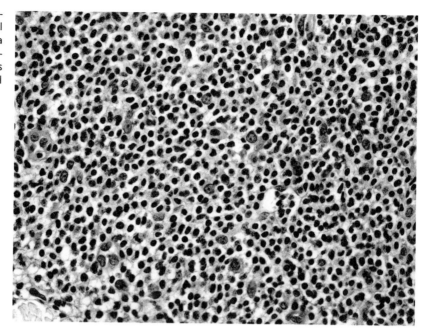

Fig. 15. Cutaneous involvement by CLL. Small lymphocytes with a round nucleus and scattered paraimmunoblasts are seen (H&E, original magnification ×40).

immunohistochemical, and molecular findings as PCMZL, and needs to be excluded clinically.

PROGNOSIS

The clinical outcome for PCMZL is excellent, with an estimated 5-year survival of 93% to 98%.[2,25–27] Solitary lesions are often treated with radiation therapy or excision, and patients with multifocal disease can get radiation therapy or a variety of systemic therapies, including rituximab.[25–27] In about half the patients, recurrences can occur after successful initial treatment but the recurrences do not necessarily appear to have a higher pathologic grade.[26] Recurrences are more common in patients who initially presented at a higher stage.[27] Rarely, patients develop systemic disease and this appears to be

Fig. 16. Cutaneous involvement by CLL. Numerous plasma cells are seen in this variant, mimicking PCMZL (H&E, original magnification ×20).

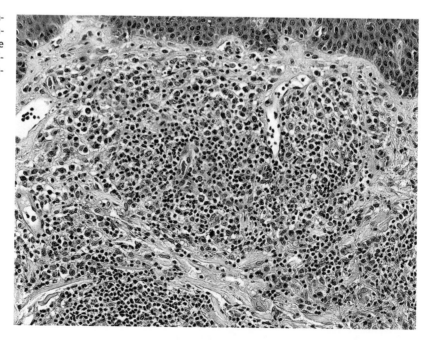

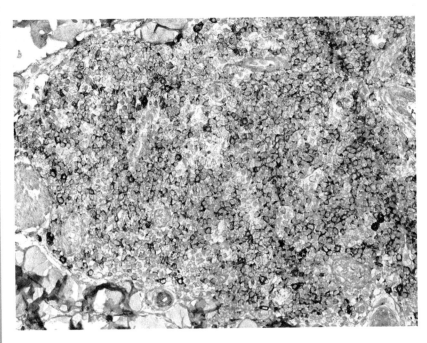

Fig. 17. Cutaneous involvement by CLL. Dim CD79a expression is seen within the small lymphocytes (original magnification ×20).

preceded in at least some cases by large-cell transformation (which is also a rare event). Death from disease is very rare. A recent study examined a series of 137 patients with PCMZL who had been treated with surgical excision, local radiotherapy, or a combination of the two. In 88% of cases, a complete remission was achieved after initial therapy, and particular success was found with solitary or localized disease.[25] However, patients

with multifocal or T3 disease showed a higher relapse rate and shorter disease-free survival, and 4% of patients developed extracutaneous disease during follow-up. Another recent study examined comorbidities that can be associated with PCMZL and found that in comparison with a control group, patients with PCMZL had a statistically significant increase in reported gastrointestinal problems, gastroesophageal reflux,

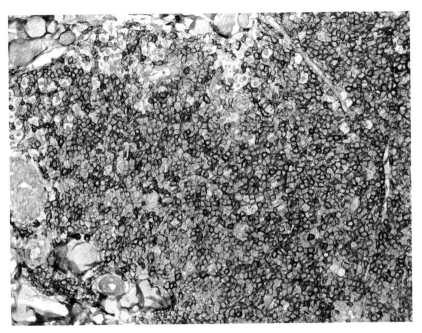

Fig. 18. Cutaneous involvement by CLL. Strong CD5 expression is seen within neoplastic B cells as well as T cells (original magnification ×20).

Fig. 19. Cutaneous involvement by chronic lymphocytic leukemia. Kappa light chain mRNA is present within lesional cells (*A*) but lambda light chain studies are negative (*B*). A, κ in situ hybridization; B, λ in situ hybridization (original magnification ×20).

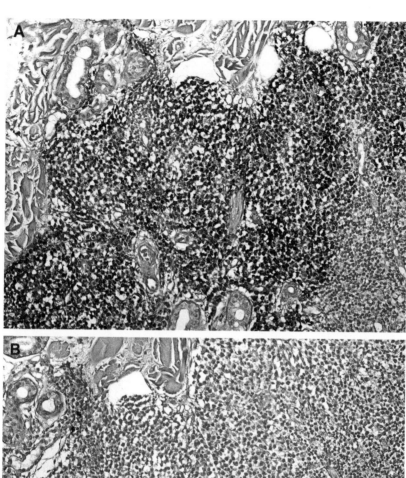

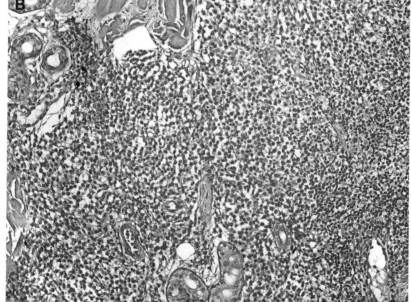

positive *Helicobacter pylori* serologies, colon disorders, autoimmune disorders, and noncutaneous malignancies.[28]

PCFCL

OVERVIEW/DEFINITION

PCFCLs are considered the most common type of PCBCL and are composed of centrocytes, centroblasts, and immunoblasts.[29] They share many of the characteristics of systemic follicular lymphomas but are skin limited at the time of presentation.

CLINICAL FEATURES

The patients are primarily adults with solitary or localized involvement of the head and neck and trunk; the scalp is a common site of involvement (**Fig. 20**). The lesions are firm plum-colored papules, plaques, or nodules. PCFCL can present as

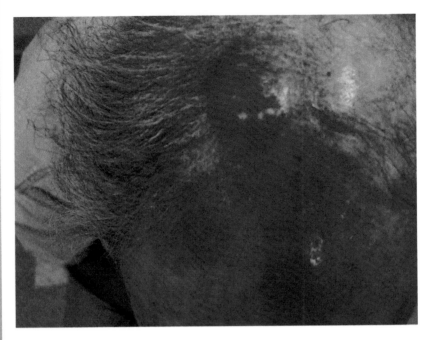

Fig. 20. PCFCL. Large erythematous nodules on the scalp of this 80-year-old man. (*Courtesy of* Youn Kim, MD, Stanford University, Stanford, CA.)

a figurate or arcuate plaque on the trunk, which is followed by development of tumors in the area, known as "reticulohistiocytoma of the dorsum" or "Crosti lymphoma."[30] Ulceration is very uncommon and presentation with multifocal disease does not predispose to a more unfavorable clinical outcome. It is thought that head and neck lesions often have a follicular pattern of involvement histologically, and Crosti lymphoma often has a diffuse pattern.[21] This entity is not thought to be significantly associated with *Borrelia burgdorferi*.

DIAGNOSIS: MICROSCOPIC FEATURES

On histology, a variety of different patterns or variants may be observed: purely follicular, follicular and diffuse, and diffuse (Box 2). The differing patterns do not confer a different prognostic outcome: rather, all 3 patterns confer an excellent clinical outcome to the patients. In the follicular variant, the infiltrate is composed of neoplastic lymphoid follicles within the dermis that contain centrocytes (cells with irregular nuclear outlines), centroblasts (enlarged cells with vesicular chromatin and prominent nucleoli), and immunoblasts (large, round cells with hyperchromatic nuclei) (Figs. 21–23). A Grenz zone is present and the epidermis is usually spared; however, rare cases with epidermotropism have been reported.[30]

Box 2
Key pathologic features of primary cutaneous follicle center lymphoma

Three patterns of involvement: follicular, mixed follicular and diffuse, and diffuse

Composed of centrocytes, centroblasts, and immunoblasts

Neoplastic follicles lack tingible body macrophages and a well-defined mantle zone

The proliferation rate, as evidenced by Ki67 and/or mib-1, is reduced in the center of neoplastic follicles

The lesional cells express CD20, CD79a, bcl-6, HGAL, and LMO2 (the latter 3 are germinal center markers); bcl-2 and CD10 are sometimes expressed

The lesional cells lack MUM1, Foxp1, IgM, and IgD

t(14;18) is not a common translocation

Light chain restriction can sometimes be demonstrated on frozen sections and in flow cytometry but is difficult to demonstrate on formalin-fixed paraffin-embedded tissues

IgH and/or IgK clonality can be demonstrated using current BIOMED-2 protocols and primers

Fig. 21. PCFCL. A dense infiltrate of lymphocytes involve the dermis in a primarily nodular pattern (H&E, original magnification ×1).

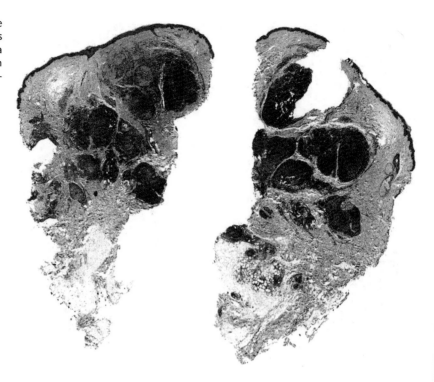

Tingible body macrophages are absent within the nodules and the mantle zone is attenuated or absent. In the follicular and diffuse variant, neoplastic follicles exist side by side with areas of more diffuse involvement by neoplastic lymphocytes. In the diffuse variant, the proliferation diffusely involves the dermis without nodular areas. All 3 patterns can extend down to involve the subcutaneous fat and can have significant amounts of centroblastic differentiation (grade III morphology). Although small lymphocytes can be numerous, eosinophils, plasma cells, and histiocytes are not commonly seen in PCFCL. A spindle-cell variant has been described.[29]

Fig. 22. PCFCL. In this high-power view of a neoplastic follicle, the mantle zone is attenuated and neoplastic centrocytes populate the center of the nodule (H&E, original magnification ×20).

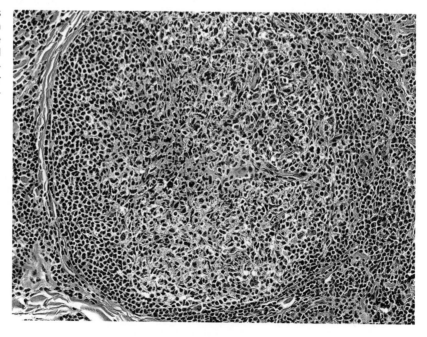

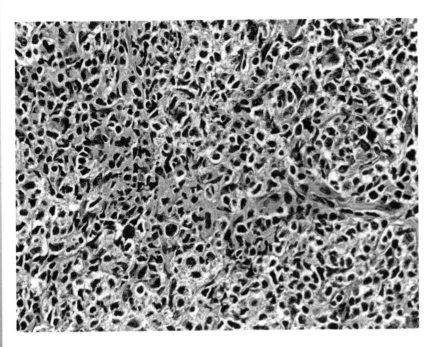

Fig. 23. PCFCL. High-power examination demonstrates numerous cells with enlarged, irregular nuclei (centrocytes) as well as larger cells with rounded nuclei (centroblasts) (H&E, original magnification ×40).

DIAGNOSIS: ANCILLARY STUDIES

On immunophenotyping, the lesional cells in all variants express CD20 and CD79a, as well as the germinal center markers bcl-6, HGAL, and LMO2 (**Fig. 24**). The bcl-6 is a transcriptional regulator required in mature B cells during germinal center processing, and is usually expressed by germinal center–derived lymphomas.[31] HGAL (GCET2, human germinal center–associated lymphoma protein) expression correlates with a favorable prognosis in patients with systemic DLBCL and classical Hodgkin lymphoma.[32] It is thought to be important for lymphocyte motility and in maintaining the structure of the germinal center and limiting the migration of germinal center–derived lymphoma cells. LMO2 (LIM domain only 2) expression also correlates with a favorable prognosis in patients with systemic DLBCL, and LMO2 is known to regulate B-cell genes implicated in kinetochore function, chromosome assembly, and mitosis.[33] Although PCFCL does express CD10 and bcl-2, similar to systemic follicular lymphomas, there is controversy in the literature regarding the amount of expression of these 2 markers. Unlike systemic follicular lymphomas, CD10 is expressed in only about 50% of the cases and bcl-2 in about 15% of the cases (usually follicular variants).[29] Diffuse expression of both of these markers should raise the possibility of secondary cutaneous involvement by systemic lymphoma. In the follicular variant, CD10 expression in lesional cells in interfollicular areas almost inevitably means that the findings are those of PCFCL. In the follicular variant and mixed follicular and diffuse variant, CD21 can be used to identify the presence of follicular dendritic cell networks (**Fig. 25**). In PCFCL, these are often associated with neoplastic cells that express germinal center markers. It is important to remember, however, that CD21 cannot be used to distinguish among PCFCL (follicular variant), PCMZL, and CLH-B. Likewise, lack of CD21 expression does not exclude the possibility of a diffuse variant of CLH-B. As expected, post–germinal center markers multiple myeloma oncogene 1 (MUM1), Forkhead box-P1 (Foxp1), IgM,[34,35] and IgD[35] are usually negative in most cases of diffuse variant of PCFCL. MUM1/interferon regulatory factor 4 (IRF4) is the product of the homologous gene involved in the multiple myeloma–associated translocation t(6;14)(p25;q32), and is expressed in the nuclei and cytoplasm of plasma cells and a small percentage of germinal center B cells.[36] Foxp1 is a winged helix transcription factor that is differentially expressed in resting and activated B cells.[37] Expression of both MUM1 and Foxp1 has been associated with poor outcome in primary cutaneous large B-cell lymphomas (PCLBCLs).[38,39] Kappa and lambda light chain restriction cannot be easily demonstrated in PCFCL and is not a useful test to support the diagnosis of lymphoma.

Fig. 24. (A–D) PCFCL. The lesional cells express the germinal center markers HGAL (A), LMO2 (B), and bcl-6 (C), but lack bcl-2 (D) (original magnification: HGAL, ×20; LMO2, ×40; bcl-6, ×60; bcl-2, ×40).

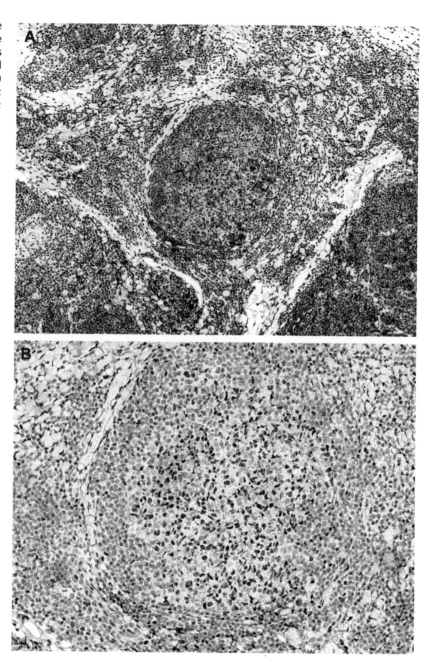

In a recent clonality study of PCFCL with BIOMED-2 protocols and primers for both *IGH* and *IGK*, monoclonality was found in all 5 cases of PCFCL tested.[40] Similarly, another study of a slightly bigger group of lymphomas found a clone in 10 of 11 cases of PCFCL using the same methods; in contrast, only 1 of 23 cases of CLH-B demonstrated a clone.[16] Detection of a clone via *IGK* analysis was higher than via *IGH* analysis, possibly due to somatic hypermutation of the latter locus.[16] t(14;18) was found very rarely in PCFCL; only 2 of 11 harbored this translocation.[16] This is in contrast to systemic follicular lymphomas, which have demonstrated t(14;18) in up to 90% of grade I to II follicular lymphomas.

DIFFERENTIAL DIAGNOSIS

For the follicular and mixed follicular and diffuse variants, the primary differential diagnostic

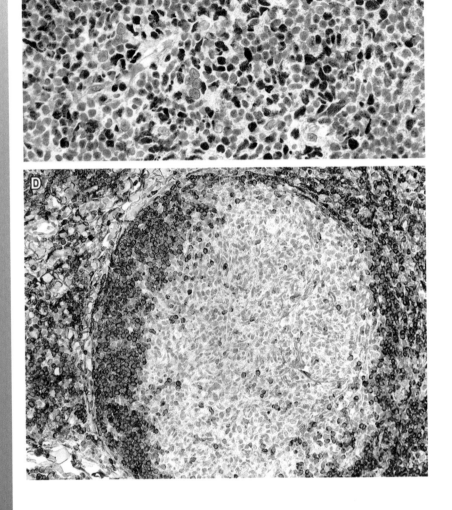

Fig. 24. (*continued*).

considerations include PCMZL and CLH-B, especially if the lesional cells are small (grade I) (see Table 1). The key difference is that PCFCL is composed of neoplastic follicles, whereas the lymphoid follicles in PCMZL are reactive. If lymphoid follicle–type structures are seen, one should look for tingible body macrophages and preservation of mantle zones; in PCFCL, tingible body macrophages and intact mantle zones are

both absent, whereas in PCMZL, both findings should be present. Similarly, in CLH-B, tingible body macrophages and intact, polarized mantle zones are present. High-power examination of the cells of PCFCL shows a large number of centrocytes, a finding that should be absent in both PCMZL and CLH-B. Lymphocytes that express CD20 and lack bcl-2 often populate the center of the lymphoid follicles of PCFCL and

Fig. 25. PCFCL. The neoplastic follicles are intimately involved with a CD21-positive follicular dendritic cell network (original magnification ×40).

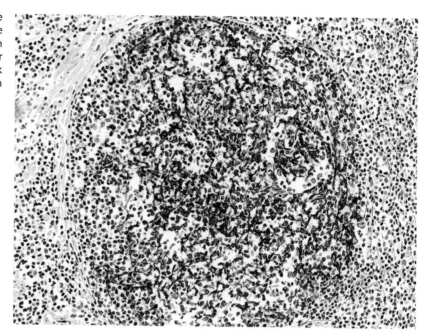

CLH-B; however, the center of a lymphoid follicle in PCMZL usually contains lymphocytes that coexpress these markers. These also lack expression of bcl-6, unlike similarly located cells in PCFCL and CLH-B. The proliferation rate (as measured by Ki67 and/or mib-1) within a lymphoid follicle of PCFCL is low (approximately 30%–40%), whereas it is often quite high in CLH-B (approximately 80%–90%).[29] The second important differential diagnostic consideration involves the diffuse variant of PCFCL and DLBCL-LT (**Box 3**). PCFCL is composed of centrocytes, centroblasts, and immunoblasts, and centrocytes tend to predominate. In DLBCL-LT, centroblasts and immunoblasts (so-called "round-cell morphology") tend to predominate. Expression of germinal center markers, such as bcl-6, CD10, HGAL, and LMO2, tend to be present in PCFCL, whereas the cells of DLBCL-LT tend to express MUM1, Foxp1, IgM, and IgD. Strong bcl-2 expression has been reported in DLBCL-LT and is thought to be a marker of poorer prognosis.[41,42] Finally, it is important to note that secondary cutaneous involvement by systemic follicular lymphoma can show identical histopathologic, immunohistochemical, and molecular findings as PCFCL, and needs to be excluded clinically. Particularly suspicious are cases that have strong expression of bcl-2 and CD10,[43] or cases of centrocyte differentiation that demonstrate expression of MUM1, Foxp1, IgM, and IgD, in addition to germinal center markers.

Box 3
Key pathologic features of primary cutaneous diffuse large B-cell lymphoma–leg type

Almost inevitably composed of a dense, diffuse, and monotonous population of large cells that extends throughout the dermis and into the subcutis

Composed of centroblasts and immunoblasts with rare centrocytes; small lymphocytes are not present

The extensive infiltrate can destroy adnexal structures

The lesional cells express CD20, CD79a, MUM1, Foxp1, IgM, and IgD; aberrant coexpression of bcl-6 (a germinal center marker) and MUM1 (an activated B-lymphocyte marker) can be a useful finding

The lesional cells lack germinal center markers, such as CD10, HGAL, and LMO2, in most cases

The bcl-2 is strongly expressed in most cases and is thought to be an independent prognostic factor

Epstein-Barr virus is negative

t(14;18) is not a common translocation

Light chain restriction can be demonstrated on formalin-fixed paraffin-embedded tissues

IgH and/or IgK clonality can be demonstrated using current BIOMED-2 protocols and primers

PROGNOSIS

PCFCL is thought to have an excellent prognosis, with a 5-year survival of 95% and higher.[29] Unlike systemic lymphomas, the outcome for patients is not dependent on growth pattern or presence or absence of t(14;18). Patients are often treated with surgery (if localized) and/or radiotherapy. Cutaneous relapses can be seen in approximately 30% of patients and is not indicative of progression (ie, systemic involvement or death). PCFCL presenting on the legs has been shown to have a poorer prognosis and have a different immunophenotypic signature.[44]

PCDLBCL-LT

OVERVIEW/DEFINITION

PCDLBCL-LT is composed of primarily centroblasts and immunoblasts, with few if any centrocytes, and arises most frequently on the legs (85%–90% of the time).[41] This is a lymphoma of intermediate prognosis, with a reported 5-year disease-specific survival of approximately 65%.[45,46]

CLINICAL FEATURES

Patients with this lymphoma are often elderly and female, and the lesions originate on the leg at presentation. The reported female-to-male ratio is 3 to 4:1 and the patients are usually older than 80.[45,46] The lesions present as tumors with a violaceous color and are often purpuric in appearance. Symmetric presentations can occur and ulceration is frequently present. Dissemination to extracutaneous sites can occur shortly after the leg lesions appear, and distinction from systemic lymphoma with secondary cutaneous involvement can be difficult. Similar lesions can occur in sites other than the leg and carry a similar clinical prognosis.[44]

DIAGNOSIS: MICROSCOPIC FEATURES

On histology, the infiltrate is composed of primarily centroblasts and immunoblasts (so-called "round-cell morphology") and involves the dermis and subcutaneous fat in a diffuse monotonous sheet (see Box 3; Figs. 26 and 27). Overlying epidermal thinning can be seen but epidermotropism is not a frequent feature. The infiltrate aggressively involves the dermis with destruction of adnexal structures. A heterogeneous infiltrate of small lymphocytes, eosinophils, plasma cells, and histiocytes is not seen.

DIAGNOSIS: ANCILLARY STUDIES

On immunophenotyping, the lesional cells express CD20 and CD79a, as well as activated B-lymphocyte markers, such as MUM1,[34,38] Foxp1,[47] IgM, and IgD (Fig. 28).[35] They usually lack expression of germinal center markers, such as HGAL[48] and CD10 (Fig. 29).[44] Conflicting reports of expression of bcl-6 have been described in the literature. Although Sundram and colleagues[38] described lack of bcl-6 in their small series of cases of PCDLBCL-LT and postulated that this may be definitional, others in larger series have not found a connection between lack of expression of bcl-6 (as a germinal center marker) and classification as PCDLBCL-LT.[39,44,47] In fact, in many of these series, bcl-6 is often expressed by PCDLBCL-LT.[46] This may be related to definitions of what constitutes PCDLBCL-LT histologically, cutoffs used to denote expression of the different immunohistochemical markers, sizes of the cohorts studied, and geographic locations of patients in the series. The bcl-2 is often strongly positive in these tumors and has been linked to prognosis.[41] In a study by Grange and colleagues,[41] 5-year disease-specific survival rates for bcl-2+ and bcl-2– tumors were 41% and 89%, respectively. Rarely, bcl-2 expression also can be seen in PCFCL, and therefore linking expression of this marker to the classification of PCDLBCL-LT should be done with caution. Ki67 and/or mib-1 can mark a significant number of these cases, but has not been shown to be important for prognosis.[38] Light chain restriction is present in a large percentage of cases.[35]

Clonality assays using the *IGH* and/or *IGK* loci are often positive; in a recent study using BIOMED-2 primers and protocols, all 6 cases tested were positive for *IGH* and/or *IGK* monoclonality.[40] Gene expression profiling of 21 cases of PCLBCLs has demonstrated increased expression of cell-cycle genes, such as *PCNA* and *CDC6*, proto-oncogenes *PIM-1*, *PIM-2*, and *c-MYC*, and transcription factors *MUM1/IRF4* and *OCT-2*.[34] Organization of these markers has revealed that expression profiling successfully divided PCLBCL into the PCFCL groups and the PCDLBCL-LT groups, respectively. In addition, there is significant evidence to suggest that PCFCL may be derived from germinal center cells and PCDLBCL-LT derived from activated B lymphocytes, similar to nodal DLBCLs. This is an important finding, as diagnostic and prognostic evaluations using immunohistochemistry can demonstrate significant variability; however, it is clear at the level of gene expression that a distinct division can be made. Some of these findings have

Fig. 26. PCDLBCL-LT. A dense diffuse infiltrate of atypical large lymphocytes involves the deep reticular dermis and subcutis (H&E, original magnification ×1).

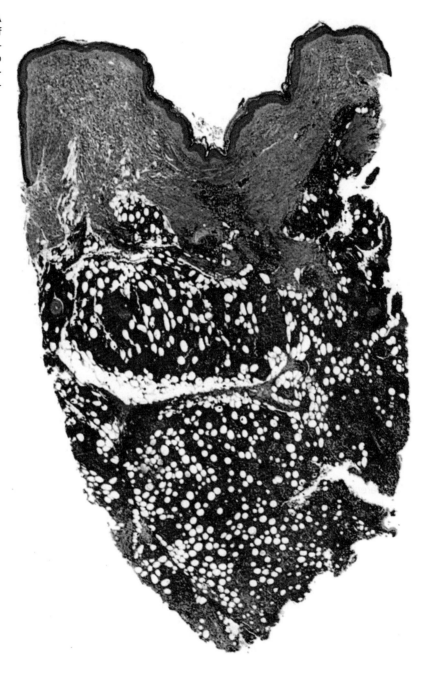

been corroborated via immunohistochemistry.[35,38,47] Interphase fluorescence in situ hybridization analysis has shown translocations involving c-MYC, BCL6, and IGH, as well as amplification of the BCL2 gene.[45] t(14;18), however, is usually absent. Analysis of somatic hypermutation in PCBCL has demonstrated aberrant somatic hypermutation in the BCL6, MYC, RhoH/TTF, and PAX5 gene loci in both PCDLBCL-LT and PCFCL, but there is higher expression of activation-induced cytidine deaminase in PCDLBCL-LT than in PCFCL at both the mRNA and protein levels.[48] Profiling of apoptosis genes only in cases of PCLBCL has demonstrated that PCDLBCL-LT is characterized by constitutive activation of the intrinsic mediated apoptosis pathway with downstream inhibition of this pathway.[49] Removal of the effects of apoptosis genes may contribute in part to the more aggressive nature of this lymphoma. Finally, deletions have been described in

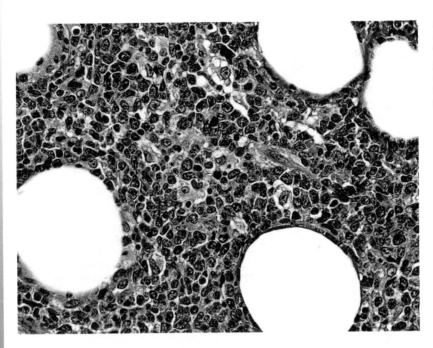

Fig. 27. PCDLBCL-LT. Higher-power view shows the infiltrate to be composed primarily of large centroblasts and immunoblasts (H&E, original magnification ×60).

the region of chromosome 9p21.3, which contains the *CDKN2A* and *CDKN2B* loci, both involved in cell cycle regulation.

DIFFERENTIAL DIAGNOSIS

The differential diagnosis of this entity should always include systemic DLBCLs with secondary cutaneous involvement, as PCDLBCL-LT is a rare entity that accounts for only 4% of all primary cutaneous lymphomas.[46] In the systemic category, considerations should include T-cell and histiocyte-rich DLBCL, CD30+ DLBCL, EBV+ DLBCL of the elderly, lymphomatoid granulomatosis, plasmablastic lymphoma, Burkitt lymphoma, intravascular large B-cell lymphoma, and DLBCL not otherwise specified. T-cell and histiocyte-rich DLBCL is very rarely primary to the skin and should be thought of as a variant of PCLBCL if a systemic workup is negative, rather than as its own entity. Cerroni and colleagues[45] have recommended, based on their own experiences, that these tumors be considered a variant of PCFCL, given their overlap in morphology to PCFCL and their overall indolent clinical behavior. Anaplastic variants of PCDLBCL-LT have been described and found to express CD30; these should be distinguished from their systemic counterparts through careful staging workups. Both lymphomatoid granulomatosis (LYG) and EBV+ DLBCL of the elderly[50] represent EBV-driven lymphoproliferative

disorders that can involve the skin as well as other extranodal sites. In the case of LYG, the skin and the lung are concomitantly involved, and patients almost always have lung lesions. Therefore, systemic workups and analysis for EBV can help distinguish these from PCDLBCL-LT. EBV+ DLBCL of the elderly is a B-cell lymphoproliferative process that is thought to arise from the natural immunosuppressed state of the elderly.[50,51] Skin, lymph node, and other extracutaneous, extranodal sites can be involved concomitantly, and skin-only presentations of this entity are uncommon. Nevertheless, sometimes the lesions can demonstrate the clinico-pathologic presentation of PCDLBCL-LT, and examination for the expression of EBV can help distinguish between this entity and PCDLBCL-LT (**Table 2**). This has important clinical implications, as EBV+ DLBCL of the elderly has a very aggressive clinical course and a median survival rate of about 2 years. Distinction from plasmablastic lymphoma can be achieved by examining the status of CD138; PCDLBCL-LT is negative for this marker. In Burkitt lymphoma, the lymphoma cells express CD38, CD43, and CD10 (in addition to B-cell markers) and have a proliferation rate of nearly 100% (as measured by Ki67 and/or mib-1). The bcl-2 is weakly positive, as opposed to the strong bcl-2 expression usually seen in PCDLBCL-LT. Finally, in intravascular large B-cell lymphomas, best considered a systemic lymphoma given frequent systemic (central

Fig. 28. (*A–E*) PCDLBCL-LT. The lesional cells express CD20 (*A*), bcl2 (*B*), IgM (*C*), Foxp1 (*D*), and MUM1 (*E*) (original magnification: CD20, ×40; bcl-2, IgM, Foxp1, MUM1 ×60).

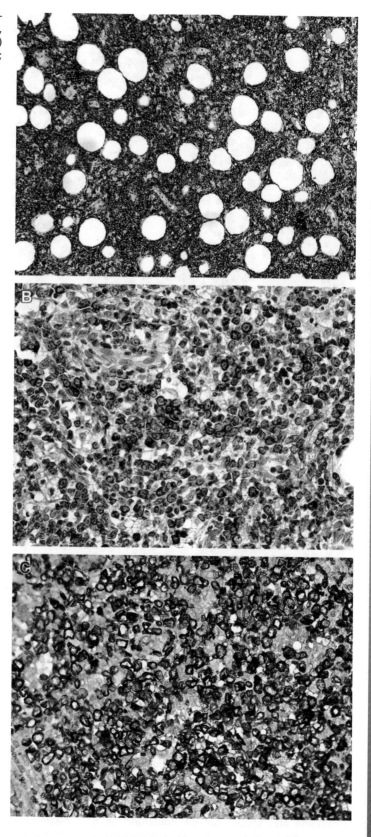

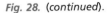

Fig. 28. (continued).

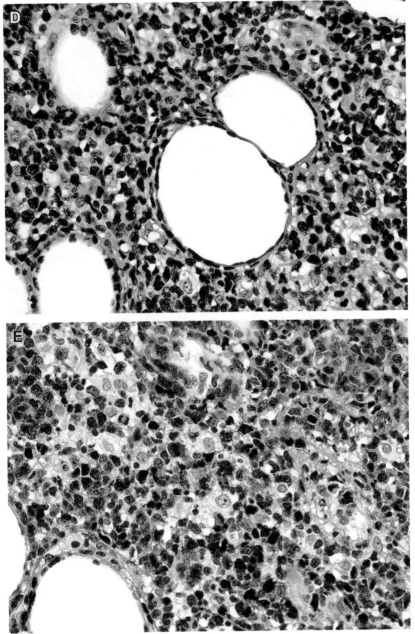

nervous system) involvement at presentation, the lymphoma cells are present intravascularly, an unusual event for PCDLBCL-LT lesions in general. However, recurrences of previously diagnosed, confirmed PCBCL can occur as an intravascular lymphoma and should not be construed as a de novo intravascular lymphoma. The distinction between PCDLBCL-LT and systemic DLBCL not otherwise specified is nearly impossible without a full systemic workup.

The most difficult differential diagnostic consideration is between PCDLBCL-LT and PCFCL. Features that favor PCFCL include centrocyte predominance (as opposed to centroblast and

Fig. 29. (A, B) PCDLBCL-LT. The lesional cells are negative for germinal center markers bcl-6 (A) and HGAL (B) (original magnification ×60).

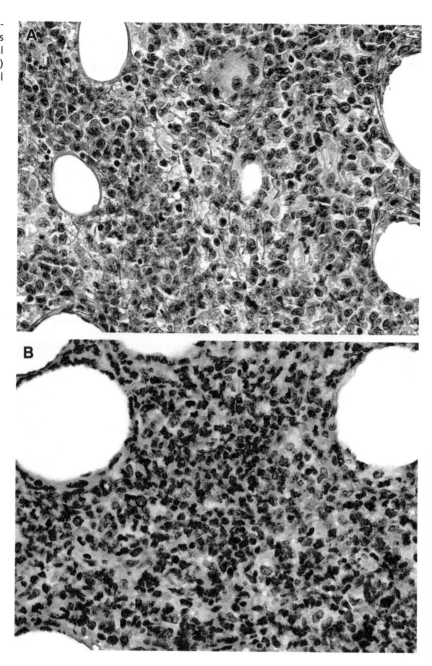

immunoblast predominance), the presence of germinal center markers, such as CD10, HGAL, and LMO2, and absence of activated B-lymphocyte markers, such as MUM1, Foxp1, IgM, and IgD. Strong bcl-2 expression and lack of expression of CD10 favors PCDLBCL-LT. The bcl-6 is difficult to use in this regard, as it is variably present in both subtypes of PCLBCL. There are reports of PCFCL arising on the legs and having a prognosis different from those arising on the head, neck, and trunk.[44] Cerroni and colleagues[21] have opined that these may in fact be PCDLBCL-LT with a centrocyte morphology and/or absence of bcl-2 and other activated B-lymphocyte

Table 2
Pathologic features that distinguish among the diffuse variant of PCFCL, PCDLBCL-LT, and EBV+ DLBCL of the elderly

	PCFCL	PCDLBCL-LT	EBV+ DLBCL of the Elderly
Patients are elderly (older than 80 y)	No	Yes	Yes
Ulceration is present	No	Yes	Yes
Lower extremity often involved	No	Yes	Yes
Centrocytes are present	Yes	No	No
Centroblasts are present	Yes	Yes	Yes
Immunoblasts are present	No	Yes	Yes
Germinal center markers are expressed (HGAL, LMO2)	Yes	No	No
Post germinal center markers are expressed (Foxp1, MUM1, IgM, IgD)	No	Yes	Yes (only the status of MUM1 is known)
EBV is expressed	No	No	Yes
Light chain restriction is present	Yes, on flow cytometry and in frozen sections	Yes	Yes
Positive IgH/IgK clonality assays	Yes	Yes	Yes

Abbreviations: DLBCL, diffuse large B-cell lymphoma; EBV, Epstein-Barr virus; Foxp1, Forkhead box-P1; Ig, immunoglobulin; MUM1, multiple myeloma oncogene 1; PCDLBCL-LT, primary cutaneous diffuse large B-cell lymphoma–leg type; PCFCL, primary cutaneous follicle center lymphoma.

markers. As it can be difficult in some cases to distinguish between these 2 entities, especially when they occur on the legs, gene expression profiling or other genomic analysis of cases such as these may shed more light on their true cell of origin.

PROGNOSIS

This lymphoma is thought to be of intermediate prognostic risk, and the presence of advanced age and multiple skin lesions at presentation are both markers of an adverse clinical outcome in multivariate analysis.[41] In addition, inactivation of CDKN2A is thought to be associated with a poorer clinical outcome. Given the aggressive nature of this lymphoma, clinicians often choose systemic chemotherapy over localized therapy such as radiation.[21] However, treatment with aggressive methods can deliver significant morbidity to the elderly patients who are primarily affected by this lymphoma. Some success has been achieved with rituximab, an anti-CD20 antibody therapy, due to its relatively benign group of side effects.

Key Features
PRIMARY CUTANEOUS B-CELL LYMPHOMAS

1. Secondary cutaneous involvement by systemic B-cell lymphoma is far more common than primary cutaneous involvement. Therefore, correlation with clinical findings and the results of imaging studies is critical to arrive at the appropriate diagnosis.

2. Key entities in this category include primary cutaneous marginal zone lymphoma (PCMZL) and its variants (immunocytoma, cutaneous plasmacytoma), primary cutaneous follicle center lymphoma (follicular and diffuse variants) (PCFCL), primary cutaneous diffuse large B-cell lymphoma–leg type, and cutaneous Epstein-Barr virus–positive diffuse large B-cell lymphoma of the elderly.

3. The distinction between primary cutaneous low-grade B-cell lymphomas (PCMZL and PCFCL, follicular variant) and B-cell–rich cutaneous lymphoid hyperplasia can be extremely difficult, even on the basis of available clinical, histopathologic, immunophenotypic, and molecular findings. Long-term clinical follow-up is essential to appropriate classification of these disorders.

Pitfalls
PRIMARY CUTANEOUS B-CELL LYMPHOMAS

! All primary cutaneous B-cell lymphomas can show morphologic and immunohistochemical features identical to those of systemic lymphomas; therefore, a complete clinical staging workup, which in some cases includes a bone marrow biopsy, has to be done in every case.

! The distinction between low-grade primary cutaneous B-cell lymphomas, such as primary cutaneous marginal zone lymphoma (PCMZL) and primary cutaneous follicle center lymphoma (PCFCL), follicular variant and B-cell rich cutaneous lymphoid hyperplasia can be quite difficult if not impossible at times: molecular studies for clonality and/or watchful waiting with repeat biopsies may aid in arriving at the appropriate diagnosis.

! Cutaneous immunocytoma and cutaneous plasmacytoma are now both considered part of PCMZL.

! PCFCL can occur as follicular variant, mixed follicular and diffuse variant, and diffuse variant: the different variants do not confer a different clinical outcome.

! CD10 and bcl-2 are rarely expressed in PCFCL, in contrast to their clinical counterparts: therefore, suspicion of secondary cutaneous involvement by systemic follicular lymphoma should be entertained whenever a cutaneous follicular lymphoma is encountered that expresses these 2 markers.

! t(14;18) is rarely expressed in PCFCL, unlike systemic follicular lymphomas or germinal center–derived diffuse large B-cell lymphoma (DLBCL).

! The distinction between PCFCL, diffuse type, and primary cutaneous diffuse large B-cell lymphoma–leg type (PCDLBCL-LT) is best done on morphologic grounds: PCFCL is composed primarily of large centrocytes with centroblasts, whereas PCDBCL-LT is composed primarily of centroblasts and immunoblasts (so-called "round-cell morphology") with few centrocytes.

! PCFCL can present primarily on the legs and these tumors are thought to have a worse clinical outcome in comparison with PCFCL occurring on the head, neck, and trunk.

! Epstein-Barr virus (EBV) is negative in PCDLBCL-LT; when EBV in situ is positive in a significant number of lesional cells, the diagnosis is more likely to be EBV+ DLBCL of the elderly.

ACKNOWLEDGMENTS

I gratefully extend my thanks to my clinical colleague, Dr Youn Kim, for providing clinical photographs, and to Norm Cyr, Stanford Pathology PhotoLab, for help with the photomicrographs within this article.

REFERENCES

1. Isaacson PG, Chott A, Nakamura S, et al. Extranodal marginal zone lymphoma of mucosa-associated lymphoid tissue (MALT lymphoma). In: Swerdlow SH, Campo E, Harris NL, et al, editors. WHO classification of tumours of haematopoietic and lymphoid tissues. Lyon (France): IARC Press; 2008. p. 214–7.

2. Cerroni L, Gatter K, Kerl H. Cutaneous marginal zone lymphoma and variants. In: Cerroni L, Gatter K, Kerl H, editors. Skin lymphoma: the illustrated guide. 3rd edition. Chichester (United Kingdom): Wiley-Blackwell Publishing; 2009. p. 141–55.

3. Hussell T, Isaacson PG, Crabtree JE, et al. The response of cells from low grade B cell gastric lymphomas of mucosa associated lymphoid tissue to Helicobacter pylori. Lancet 1993;342:571–4.

4. Goodlad JR, Davidson MM, Hollowood K, et al. Primary cutaneous B cell lymphoma and Borrelia burgdorferi infection in patients from the highlands of Scotland. Am J Surg Pathol 2000;24:1279–85.

5. Rijlaarsdam JU, van der Putte SC, Berti E, et al. Cutaneous immunocytomas: a clinicopathologic study of 26 cases. Histopathology 1993;23: 117–25.

6. LeBoit PE, McNutt NS, Reed JA, et al. Primary cutaneous immunocytoma: a B cell lymphoma that can easily be mistaken for cutaneous lymphoid hyperplasia. Am J Surg Pathol 1994;18:969–78.

7. Magro CM, Porcu P, Ahmad N, et al. Cutaneous immunocytoma: a clinical, histologic, and phenotypic study of 11 cases. Appl Immunohistochem Mol Morphol 2004;12:216–24.

8. Lee BA, Jacobson M, Seidel G. Epidermotropic marginal zone lymphoma simulating mycosis fungoides. J Cutan Pathol 2013;40:569–72.

9. Tsuji K, Suzuki D, Naito Y, et al. Primary cutaneous marginal zone B-cell lymphoma. Eur J Dermatol 2005;15:480–3.

10. de la Fouchardière A, Balme B, Chouvet B, et al. Primary cutaneous marginal zone B-cell lymphoma: a report of 9 cases. J Am Acad Dermatol 1999;41:181–8.

11. Baldassano MF, Bailey EM, Ferry JA, et al. Cutaneous lymphoid hyperplasia and cutaneous marginal zone lymphoma: comparison of morphologic and immunophenotypic features. Am J Surg Pathol 1999;23:88–96.

12. Magro C. The expression of CD23 and CD40 in primary cutaneous B-cell lymphomas. J Cutan Pathol 2007;34:461–6.

13. Levin C, Mirzamani N, Zwerner J, et al. A comparative analysis of cutaneous marginal zone lymphoma and cutaneous chronic lymphocytic leukemia. Am J Dermatopathol 2012;34:18–23.

14. Magro C, Crowson AN, Porcu P, et al. Automated kappa and lambda light chain mRNA expression for the assessment of B cell clonality in cutaneous B-cell infiltrates: its utility and diagnostic application. J Cutan Pathol 2003;30:504–11.

15. Kutzner H, Kerl H, Pfaltz MC, et al. CD123-positive plasmacytoid dendritic cells in primary cutaneous marginal zone B cell lymphoma: diagnostic and pathogenetic implications. Am J Surg Pathol 2009;33:1307–13.

16. Morales AV, Arber DA, Seo K, et al. Evaluation of B cell clonality using the BIOMED-2 PCR method effectively distinguishes cutaneous B cell lymphoma from benign lymphoid infiltrates. Am J Dermatopathol 2008;30:425–30.

17. Fujiwara M, Morales AV, Seo K, et al. Clonal identity and differences in primary cutaneous B cell lymphoma occurring at different sites or time points in the same patient. Am J Dermatopathol 2013; 35:11–8.

18. Gallardo F, Bellosillo B, Espinet B, et al. Aberrant nuclear BCL10 expression and lack of t(11;18)(q21;q21) in primary cutaneous marginal zone B-cell lymphoma. Hum Pathol 2006;37: 867–73.

19. de la Fouchardiere A, Gazzo S, Balme B, et al. Cytogenetic and molecular analysis of 12 cases of primary cutaneous marginal zone lymphoma. Am J Dermatopathol 2006;28:287–92.

20. Cerroni L, Zenahlik P, Hofler G, et al. Specific cutaneous infiltrates of B-cell chronic lymphocytic leukemia: a clinicopathologic and prognostic study of 42 patients. Am J Surg Pathol 1996;20:1000–10.

21. Cerroni L, Gatter K, Kerl H. Cutaneous follicle center lymphoma. In: Cerroni L, Gatter K, Kerl H, editors. Skin lymphoma: the illustrated guide. 3rd edition. Chichester (United Kingdom): Wiley-Blackwell Publishing; 2009. p. 129–40.

22. de Leval L, Harris NL, Longtine J, et al. Cutaneous B cell lymphomas of follicular and marginal zone types. Use of bcl-6, bcl-2, and CD21 in differential diagnosis and classification. Am J Surg Pathol 2001;25:732–41.

23. Jayaraman AG, Cesca C, Kohler S. Cutaneous plasmacytosis. A report of five cases with immunohistochemical evaluation for HHV-8 expression. Am J Dermatopathol 2006;28:93–8.

24. Tomasini D, Zampatti C, Serio G. Castleman's disease with numerous mantle zone lymphocytes with clear cytoplasm involving the skin: case report. J Cutan Pathol 2009;36:887–91.

25. Servitje O, Muniesa C, Benavente Y, et al. Primary cutaneous marginal zone B cell lymphoma: response to treatment and disease free survival in a series of 137 patients. J Am Acad Dermatol 2013;69:357–65.

26. Hoefnagel JJ, Vermeer MH, Jansen PM, et al. Primary cutaneous marginal zone B cell lymphoma: clinical and therapeutic features in 50 cases. Arch Dermatol 2005;141:1139–45.

27. Gerami P, Wickless SC, Rosen S, et al. Applying the new TNM classification system for primary cutaneous lymphomas other than mycosis fungoides and Sézary syndrome in primary cutaneous marginal zone lymphoma. J Am Acad Dermatol 2008; 59:245–54.

28. Guitart J, Deonisio J, Bloom T, et al. High incidence of gastrointestinal tract disorders and autoimmunity in primary cutaneous marginal zone B-cell lymphomas. JAMA Dermatol 2014. http://dx.doi.org/10.1001/jamadermatol.2013.9233.

29. Willemze R, Swerdlow SH, Harris NL, et al. Primary cutaneous follicle centre lymphoma. In: Swerdlow SH, Campo E, Harris NL, et al, editors. WHO classification of tumours of haematopoietic and lymphoid tissues. Lyon (France): IARC Press; 2008. p. 227–8.

30. Plaza JA, Kacerovska D, Stockman DL, et al. The histomorphologic spectrum of primary cutaneous diffuse large B cell lymphoma: a study of 79 cases. Am J Dermatopathol 2011;33:649–55.

31. Basso K, Dalla-Favera R. Roles of BCL6 in normal and transformed germinal center B cells. Immunol Rev 2012;247:172–83.

32. Lu X, Chen J, Malumbres R, et al. HGAL, a lymphoma prognostic biomarker, interacts with the cytoskeleton and mediates the effects of IL-6 on cell migration. Blood 2007;110:4268–77.

33. Cubedo E, Gentles AJ, Huang C, et al. Identification of LMO2 transcriptome and interactome in diffuse large B cell lymphoma. Blood 2012;119:5478–91.

34. Hoefnagel JJ, Dijkman R, Basso K, et al. Distinct expression of primary cutaneous large B cell lymphoma identified by gene expression profiling. Blood 2005;105:3671–8.

35. Koens L, Vermeer MH, Willemze R, et al. IgM expression on paraffin sections distinguishes primary cutaneous large B cell lymphoma, leg type from primary cutaneous follicle center lymphoma. Am J Surg Pathol 2010;34:1043–8.

36. Falini B, Fizzotti M, Pucciarini A, et al. A monoclonal antibody (MUM1p) detects expression of the MUM1/IRF4 protein in a subset of germinal center B cells, plasma cells, and activated T cells. Blood 2000;95:2084–92.

37. Barrans SL, Fenton JA, Banham A, et al. Strong expression of FOXP1 identifies a distinct subset of diffuse large B cell lymphoma (DLBCL) patients with poor outcome. Blood 2004;104:2933–5.

38. Sundram U, Kim Y, Mraz-Gernhard S, et al. Expression of the bcl-6 and MUM1/IRF4 proteins correlate with overall and disease-specific survival in patients with primary cutaneous large B cell lymphoma: a tissue microarray study. J Cutan Pathol 2005;32:227–34.

39. Kodama K, Massone C, Chott A, et al. Primary cutaneous large B cell lymphomas: clinicopathologic features, classification, and prognostic factors in a large series of patients. Blood 2005;106: 2491–7.

40. Felcht M, Booken N, Stroebel P, et al. The value of molecular diagnostics in primary cutaneous B cell lymphomas in the context of clinical findings, histology, and immunohistochemistry. J Am Acad Dermatol 2011;64:135–43.

41. Grange F, Petrella T, Beylot-Barry M, et al. Bcl-2 protein expression is the strongest independent prognostic factor of survival in primary cutaneous large B cell lymphomas. Blood 2004;103:3662–8.

42. Grange F, Beylot-Barry M, Courville P, et al. Primary cutaneous diffuse large B cell lymphoma, leg type: clinicopathologic features and prognostic analysis in 60 cases. Arch Dermatol 2007;143:1144–50.

43. Kim BK, Surti U, Pandya AG, et al. Primary and secondary cutaneous diffuse large B cell lymphomas. A multiparameter analysis of 25 cases including fluorescence in situ hybridization for t(14;18) translocation. Am J Surg Pathol 2003;27: 356–64.

44. Senff NJ, Hoefnagel JJ, Jansen PM, et al. Reclassification of 300 primary cutaneous B cell lymphomas according to the new WHO-EORTC classification for cutaneous lymphomas: comparison with previous classifications and identification of prognostic markers. J Clin Oncol 2007;25: 1581–7.

45. Cerroni L, Gatter K, Kerl H. Cutaneous diffuse large B cell lymphoma, leg type. In: Cerroni L, Gatter K, Kerl H, editors. Skin lymphoma: the illustrated guide. 3rd edition. Chichester (United Kingdom): Wiley-Blackwell Publishing; 2009. p. 156–63.

46. Meijer CJ, Vergier B, Duncan LM, et al. Primary cutaneous DLBCL, leg type. In: Swerdlow SH, Campo E, Harris NL, et al, editors. WHO classification of tumours of haematopoietic and lymphoid tissues. Lyon (France): IARC Press; 2008. p. 242.

47. Hoefnagel JJ, Mulder MM, Dreef E, et al. Expression of B cell transcription factors in primary cutaneous B cell lymphomas. Mod Pathol 2006;19: 1270–6.

48. Djikman R, Tensen CP, Buettner M, et al. Primary cutaneous follicle center lymphoma and primary cutaneous large B cell lymphoma, leg type, are both targeted by aberrant somatic hypermutation but demonstrate differential expression of AID. Blood 2006;107:4926–9.

49. van Galen JC, Hoefnagel JJ, Vermeer MH, et al. Profiling of apoptosis genes identifies distinct types of primary cutaneous large B cell lymphoma. J Pathol 2008;215:340–6.

50. Montes-Moreno S, Odqvist L, Diaz-Perez JA, et al. EBV positive diffuse large B cell lymphoma of the elderly is an aggressive post germinal center B cell neoplasm characterized by prominent nuclear factor-κB activation. Mod Pathol 2012;25:968–82.

51. Suarez AL, Querfeld C, Horwitz S, et al. Primary cutaneous B cell lymphomas. Part II. Therapy and future directions. J Am Acad Dermatol 2013;343: e1–11.

Index

Note: Page numbers of article titles are in **boldface** type.

Surgical Pathology 7 (2014) 285–289
http://dx.doi.org/10.1016/S1875-9181(14)00031-2
1875-9181/14/$ – see front matter © 2014 Elsevier Inc. All rights reserved.

Moving?

Make sure your subscription moves with you!

To notify us of your new address, find your **Clinics Account Number** (located on your mailing label above your name), and contact customer service at:

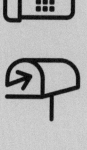

Email: journalscustomerservice-usa@elsevier.com

800-654-2452 (subscribers in the U.S. & Canada)
314-447-8871 (subscribers outside of the U.S. & Canada)

Fax number: 314-447-8029

Elsevier Health Sciences Division
Subscription Customer Service
3251 Riverport Lane
Maryland Heights, MO 63043

*To ensure uninterrupted delivery of your subscription, please notify us at least 4 weeks in advance of move.

ELSEVIER

Printed and bound by CPI Group (UK) Ltd, Croydon, CR0 4YY

03/10/2024

01040378-0016